KARL LAGERFELD
DIET

Karl Lagerfeld was born in Hamburg in 1936. He is a clothes designer, photographer, bookseller, publisher, and gallery owner. In 1996 he was awarded the Culture Prize by the German Society of Photography (Deutsche Gesellschaft für Photographie).

Jean-Claude Houdret is a general practitioner, specializing in nutrition, aesthetics, herbal medicine, and homeopathy. He teaches medicine at the University of Paris 13 and is the author of several works. He lives and works in Paris.

Ingrid Sischy is editor of *Interview* magazine in New York.

"You can go from oversized to the size dictated by either fashion or your own desires. For that you need a doctor, not necessarily a designer, but you do have to go on a diet...."
—Karl Lagerfeld

THE
KARL LAGERFELD
DIET

Karl Lagerfeld and
Jean-Claude Houdret

Interview by Ingrid Sischy

 powerHouse Books New York, NY

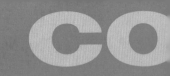

ntents

Slim, attractive, and fit 169

Conclusion by Jean-Claude Houdret 213

Tables 217

Postscript by Jean-Claude Houdret 219

Index of recipes 221

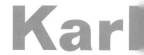

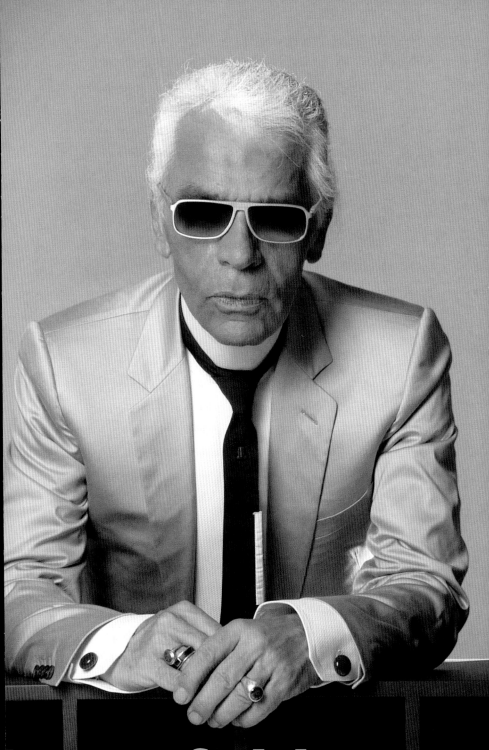

Lagerfeld

Merci cher ami

pour tous ces jolis papillons.

Bises Jean

13.x.02

Foreword

How can we discover our "true nature," our "inner being," if we have not experimented with different ways of being? If you attach no importance to weight problems, if not being able to wear new, trendy small-sized clothes does not cause you any regret, this book is not for you. Health reasons are an excellent motive for losing weight and for some they are truly vital. But if you are lucky enough not to need to go on a diet for such reasons, there is nothing to stop you from pretending to others that health is indeed your motivation, in order to avoid having to explain to them that your true, deeper motives have nothing to do with health. In one sense, mental health is even more important. Above all you must be convinced of your ability to succeed. There is no hurry. You have no deadline for a new life!

Off you go, throw yourself into it, follow your doctor's advice and tell yourself that it is essential—even if it isn't. Take things seriously—but without making them all-important. Treat the "cleansing isolation" that a rigorous diet entails as an interesting experience. Don't do it just in order to change your life or, worse, because of a new love. These are poor reasons, that could lead you straight to depression. This is a question of your own happiness—others come or don't come later. At first your closest friends (or lovers) should not even know that you have decided to make yourself over. You will have plenty of time to discuss it later but, to begin with, it must be a secret pact with yourself. "Beauty"—or the desire to be beautiful—is in itself a dangerous motivation. Someone (I forget who) once said, "Does the person who loves someone for their beauty really love them?" So don't focus on beauty—while recognizing that the idea has crossed your mind. A respectable appearance is sufficient to make people more interested in your soul. It is the sum of our experiences that makes us interesting and having been through a time in your life, in which you were in a bad place (or what you perceived as a bad place) physically, can be useful. It can even be necessary. In any case, once on the downward slope, "perfect and pure beauty" never retraces its steps.

Concern for your appearance can help you retain your fitness or even increase it. There comes a moment in life when the idea of youth and beauty has to give way to style and elegance. That's how it is. The gaze of youth is pitiless. Do you recall what you thought, at the age of twenty, of anyone over thirty? Everyone is the same. Impress young people with what they cannot hope to be at their age. They may think that is unimportant, but age encourages indulgence. Youth is a club from which all the members will eventually end up being excluded. Don't try to compete with the young. If they have any sense, they will realize that their membership in this club is finite. But, at the same time, don't forget that youth has nothing to do with the spiritual beauty of older people. If you are over thirty-five, don't set yourself up to be compared with young people: rather, try to find something in yourself that they will be able to use as an example when their time comes to be expelled from the "paradise" of youth.

What we are depends on circumstance, but make use of yourself the way a painter makes use of his model. Imagine that you are an actor looking for new roles. Start your diet during a period of optimism and happiness. You will have to detach yourself from your physical being for a period of time and you will need to regard your social environment as unimportant. Right from the start you must devote all your energies to your diet. It is an exclusively physical regimen, so it is better to see your diet as such rather than in psychological terms (which is not easy). You will need to adopt a sort of double life. Don't talk about it too much. One's diet is as boring a subject of conversation as illness! Fitness is as boring as sickness.

After this diet you may feel that you have rediscovered a sort of second youth. Although it will obviously not be on a par with the first, it will nevertheless prove to be extremely pleasant if you modify your priorities. Avoid literary psychology—that has no place in this diet. It is merely a question of putting distance between yourself and someone you no longer love, with whom you no longer wish to share a body....

You may have immediate goals in mind, but don't expect immediate results. Be pragmatic and long term in your goals. We are talking about a process that is sometimes very "realistic"; almost mundane. The only words that can make you lose weight are those pronounced by your doctor: the rules of your diet. Remember that games, too, have rules. Winning the game…that will be your favorite diet.

Karl Lagerfeld

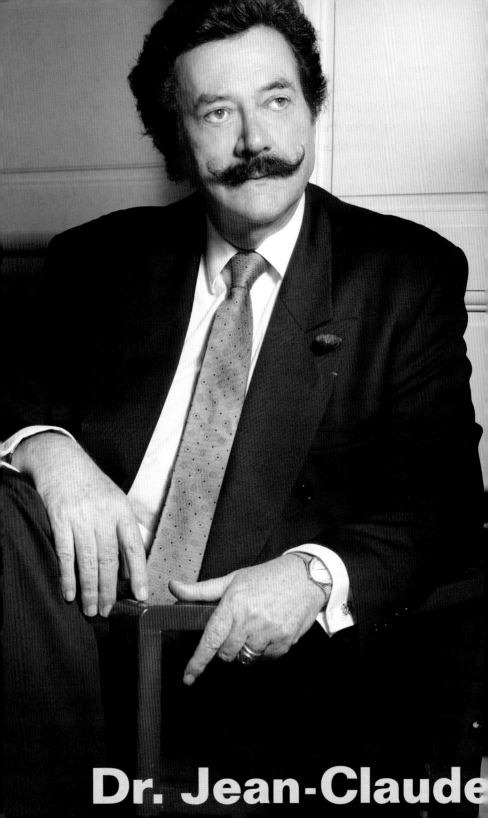

Dr. Jean-Claude

Foreword

Behind the apparent frivolity of the subject of "how and why a great couturier lost more than 80 pounds" there hides a very serious problem in society: obesity is becoming widespread in the world and in the coming decades will constitute the principal cause of death (not directly, but indirectly through its complications: diabetes and its consequences, high blood pressure, mobility problems, respiratory problems, etc.).

If famine was a scourge for humanity in the still-recent past, I think that overeating will be a scourge for humanity in the future. It is sugar, above all, that is the problem, as there has been an exponential rise in its consumption. As soon as people emerge from extreme poverty and undernourishment and are brutally thrown into the consumer society where there is easy access to abundant food, they throw themselves on sweet foods in a frenzy, as if sugar were the new opium of the masses to make them forget their pain and suffering.

The fact that this is the same in every industrialized country in the world confirms that the taste for sugar is universal.

This is a societal rather than a strictly medical problem. As with smoking, it is well known that sugar abuse is dangerous and that society at large will have to bear the cost of the resulting illnesses. So the real question is, how can we protect individuals from themselves, and how can we protect society from the excesses of individuals?

At a time when the number of obese children is rising relentlessly in the United States, England, Germany, France, and throughout the Western world, when permissiveness is rising, and when—in the name of tolerance and the right of each person to be what he wants to be—it is more and more forbidden to forbid, the future of anti-obesity measures is unclear to say the least.

Karl Largerfeld's case is emblematic and spectacular as it demonstrates the possibility, through determination and willpower, of returning to a harmonious balance even when excess weight is of a long-standing, deeply ingrained nature.

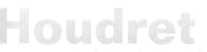

I hope that many will be inspired by the example of the slimmed-down, elegant, and indefatigable Karl Lagerfeld to lose either the few pounds they feel should be sacrificed for their happiness or the several dozen pounds that they must lose for their health.

Jean-Claude Houdret

Dieting is the only game where you **win** when you lose

Interview between Ingrid Sischy and Karl Lagerfeld

INGRID SISCHY: Now, Karl, tell us how this diet started.

KARL LAGERFELD: One fine morning I woke up and decided that I was no longer happy with my physique. I had gotten along fine with being overweight and had no health problems, but I suddenly wanted to dress differently, to wear clothes designed by Hedi Slimane, who used to work for Saint Laurent and now creates the Dior Homme collections. But these fashions, modeled by very, very slim boys (and not men of my age) would require me to lose at least 80 pounds.

On November 1, 2000, when I started my diet, I did not think that it was possible to lose so much weight in one year—to tell the truth, that was because I didn't expect it to last so long. In fact, it took me exactly thirteen months. So I started that day without a precise time frame in mind, following the advice of my doctor, Jean-Claude Houdret. And now here we are writing a book about the diet. I would never have thought it possible to achieve this result without feeling the least bit tired. Today, however, I work better than ever and I am never tired. I have seven undisturbed hours of sleep a night—and without using sleeping pills. People imagine that I needed iron willpower and discipline. I don't think so. I had decided to become a perfect clotheshorse of 132 pounds (for a height of five foot eleven), the weight necessary to wear the new tailored look, and to get the appropriate physique. I had already begun to limit my purchases from Japanese designers—I had seen a bit too much of their ample, oversized designs and was tired of wearing them. They had given me good and loyal service over many years—I felt well dressed, modern, and smart. I had liked the materials and the concept of these clothes very much. I had been wearing them for more than ten years—my black period—and can't say that I was unhappy with them. It was myself I was no longer satisfied with. I was starting to say to myself, "You work in fashion and fashion means change. If you don't like your image, you only have to change it. It's not a matter of going back to what you used to be." So it was for totally superficial reasons that I got started on this diet. That idea does not disturb me. I think that, for women as well as for men, fashion is the healthiest motivation for losing weight. It was a matter of clothes. I had no health problems nor—which would be worse—emotional problems! It is not a good idea to wait until you are ill or unhappy to go on a diet. I wasn't suffering from high blood pressure. I weighed too much, of course, but that is something entirely relative—it all depends on how you feel. I wasn't really giving in to a narcissistic impulse, either. It was time for a change, that was all. Moreover, I have forgotten the man I was two years ago, I can't remember him.

I couldn't tell you in precise detail what pushed me to go on a diet. For my professional credibility, it is a good thing to be able to prove that I am capable of creating transformations—not only my designs but also my own appearance. The boots, the shirts, the black trousers—the whole package—represented a sort of camouflage. It worked perfectly and I have to say that I lived very well in those outfits—or rather behind them. The dark glasses, the fan—they were like a wall between the world and myself. Then I said to myself, "What if I had a glass wall so that I could see through it better?" Of course, by seeing through it better I am also exposing myself more to view. Now that I have finished my diet, I still have the same friends and I do the same things as before.

IS: What sort of man were you at thirty? Very athletic, to judge by the photos of the time.

KL: In the photos taken at Saint-Tropez with the illustrator Antonio Lopez and all those bodybuilders I was barely thirty. But there is another me that few people have ever seen. The eighteen-, nineteen-, and twenty-year-old me.

IS: Can you tell me about it?

KL: I was still in school when I moved to Paris. But it didn't take me long to discover that the essential thing in life—I'm talking about the fifties—was to be well dressed. My father was obviously not going to spend crazy amounts on frivolities, he wasn't the type to throw money out the window, but he belonged to a generation that attached great importance to one's style of dress. He used to say that if you arrived at the office well dressed, half the work was done. So he was not against the idea of made-to-measure shirts, elegant suits, and fine shoes. At that time everything had to be ordered. You couldn't find many nice things in the shops. When I first became interested in fashion there was a shop in Paris called Eddi, which was in the Galerie du Lido on the Champs-Elysées. There was also a famous café where everyone went to eat hamburgers at lunchtime and after midnight. I used to go there too, and do a little shopping afterwards. It was a fairly stylish place and seeing all those clothes—and all those stylish people doing their shopping—I said to myself that the moment had possibly come for me to move on to made-to-measure suits. I must have been sixteen or seventeen, and I tried very tactfully to persuade my father. It wasn't all that easy because I didn't want to go to his German tailor (who was perfect for him, incidentally). I wanted Cifonelli, the Italian tailor who was the darling of Paris at the time. I wanted him and only him.

IS: **Had you already started work? Or were you still a student?**

KL: No, I was working for Balmain. I was seventeen and just starting out. There was one day I shall never forget. It was during the winter of 1956, the coldest Paris winter in living memory. My father was staying at the Georges V, where he always stayed when he was in Paris. It was a very comfortable hotel but I wasn't allowed to stay there because my parents felt that it was unsuitable for a young man. They were frightened of letting me think that life was too easy, and there were too many temptations that they preferred not to put in the path of a young man. So I went to visit my father—it was a winter's day; too cold even for snow and I was not wearing a coat. My father said, "But you aren't wearing a coat!" "No," I replied. "But you have loads of them," he insisted. I explained to him that I had given them away. "But why? Are you crazy?" "No, no, not at all," I answered. "Just across from the hotel there is a shop called Dorian Gray. They have a navy blue, cashmere overcoat, cut like a dressing gown. I want it. And if I can't have it I would prefer to die of cold." I said to my father that I would not wear any other coat; that I would stay in bed and not go out. If he wanted me to go out, I absolutely had to have it. So he crossed the street and bought it for me.

IS: Well done, Karl! And what type of body did you have at the time? And what was your style?

KL: I was very, very thin but I wanted to have broader shoulders. I weighed the same as today. For a while I had fairly short hair. As a child I had always worn it long but I had it cut because I felt that was the thing to do in the 1950s. So my father said to me, "Go and have some shirts made at Hilditch & Key. I'll buy you a few suits at Cifonelli and you can order yourself some shoes at Hellstern." That's how I got my first Hilditch shirt. I became one of their best clients in the whole world and I still go there today. I'm like the women who order haute couture dresses. When I buy, I really go for it. I am crazy about shirts. If you asked me what I would have preferred to have invented in the world of fashion I would answer the white shirt. For me a shirt is the basis of everything—everything else follows after. The greatest moment in life for a man is when he is getting dressed in the morning and he puts on a clean, well-ironed shirt.

IS: So your father appreciated elegance?

KL: Yes, he had his personal tailor in Germany—Staben in Hamburg. When I was fourteen, this tailor made me a suit in salt-and-pepper grey with my first long trousers, but I didn't like it. At the end of his life, when he was nearly ninety, my father only wore pale colors, pale grey—grey hats, grey suits with white shirts, and grey ties decorated with a pearl. It was perfect with his grey hair. I found him very elegant. But I don't look like him at all. I have a completely different body shape.

IS: Was your father slim?

KL: Yes. Perhaps not that year, but he always had a slender but still robust figure, even at the age of ninety. Between fifty and sixty he was a little rounder but still well built. He had a short upper body and long legs. I have the opposite problem. I wouldn't say my legs are short but they're not really long, either. I don't find my short legs particularly elegant but I have always appreciated their thin shape and my lack of hips. I get that from my mother.

IS: When you were young, were you always impeccably dressed?

KL: Yes. My mother and father were very well groomed. They always said that there is nothing worse than to be casually dressed when you are past the first flush of youth. When you are young you can get away with it but once you are over twenty-five you have to be more careful, and over thirty, well...I was born to be impeccably turned out and they always encouraged me to be so.

IS: Judging by the photos of the time you were rather a good-looking young man, very glamorous.

KL: That's a word which would never have been used to describe a man at the time. There aren't many people left who could tell you about those days. I hadn't really started work at that time—I used to go out in the evening and go dancing until five or six in the morning. I would leave the nightclub to go directly to the fashion houses of Balmain or Patou. Don't forget that at the end of the 1950s when you went out dancing it was to dance, not to take drugs or to go drinking.

IS: And in your opinion, at what stage did you lose this perfect body, this very *soigné* appearance that looked good in everything?

KL: At the beginning of the 1960s that look went out of fashion. It was too elegant. But at the Renoma brothers' shop in the rue de la Pompe, they made clothes with narrow shoulders and a completely different cut intended for very thin men. The trendy young things of the time, whom everyone was talking about, such as Jacques Dutronc and Johnny Hallyday, were very slim and you needed to look like them to wear the clothes. But after a few years I got tired of them too. Then I let myself be talked into bodybuilding by a friend. It wasn't really in style at the end of the 1960s but I was thirty and I told myself that it might be a good idea. It looked good on the beach and it fit the look I liked. So I started to do it and I enjoyed it. Then I went back to Cifonelli because a bodybuilder needs clothes that are very well made but also reasonably generously cut. Those little figure-hugging outfits didn't look good on me any more. I had had enough of them.

IS: Did you have weight-lifting equipment at home?

KL: Oh, no. I used to go to a club in the eighth arrondissement for three hours at a time, at least four times a week. All the elegant gigolos of the time used to meet there in the afternoons. They had to watch their figure in order to please their clients. It's funny, isn't it? It wasn't just a gay world, though—these "kept" boys were not homosexuals. Perhaps a few were but in general, if a client was prepared to pay for a boy, he didn't want to compete with other men. It didn't matter to him if he saw the boy with a girl in the evening—the gigolos met their clients at lunchtime. But he couldn't bear the thought that a boy he was with might be thinking about another man. So as soon as a gigolo had an affair with a man—which could happen—he had to be really discreet because, if his client found out, he would be sure to be dropped. It was the opposite of that famous late-nineteenth-century novel, *Monsieur Vénus*, by Rachilde. A Visconti-type situation.

IS: Life seems so boring today in comparison.

KL: You should never make comparisons. I knew all those gigolos but I was not one of them. Still, this did not prevent one of my former assistants, who was eighteen at the time, from being convinced of the opposite. I was young, I drove a Bentley and I was much better dressed than many others. He obviously wondered how I could afford to pay for all that. Since I frequented the world of gigolos, he must have thought that I was quite a successful one myself!

IS: **Did everyone go to the gym during the day?**

KL: Yes, the best time was the afternoon. I wasn't ambitious back then. I didn't put much effort into anything but weight lifting.

IS: **All the same, Karl, you were already working for all the big fashion houses.**

KL: Yes, but I wasn't working all that much. I was working for Chloé and Fendi, but there were two collections for Chloé and one for Fendi, of just fur! I was working even less for Krizia. I also worked for Charles Jourdan but that still left me plenty of time for everything else.

IS: **You obviously haven't changed. You have always given the impression of managing to fit in more than anyone else. But tell me, did bodybuilding and the world of fashion at that time work well together?**

KL: At the end of the 1960s I went back to Cifonelli because I had an athletic body of the type you see a lot today. It was fairly rare at the time and Cifonelli's clothes fit me perfectly. One day in '72 or '73 I went to Cifonelli for a fitting and M. Cifonelli—a very small man—asked me, "Could you come back this afternoon, I'm rather tired." And by the afternoon he was dead. What a tragedy, he was such a genius. His nephew took over the business but the clothes didn't hang on me like before. From then on I had my clothes made to measure by a tailor, according to my own sketches.

IS: **Did that enable you to get the designs you wanted?**

KL: Yes. That tailor followed my designs exactly. Then one day, in the early 1970s, I think, I was at the gym and I realized that it bored me to death. I stopped. You have to devote yourself wholeheartedly to that type of thing; otherwise it doesn't work. I started to put on weight. I invented an item of clothing called the "over-blouse"—it was a very loosely cut shirt with a scarf over a second shirt. I layered scarves and over-blouses on top of each other. Everybody started to wear them—

Jackie Onassis, Antonio, Julien Clerc, whom I used to dress at that time, everybody.

IS: You invented this item of clothing because you had put on weight?

KL: Of course. But I still wasn't fat. Then suddenly, in about 1978, I got tired of the bohemian look and all its improvisations. I was also fed up with going goodness knows how many times to that tailor to try on the same suit, which never fit. I had other things to do. I had more work and I wanted to go to Caraceni in Milan. They made fantastic clothes for me there. I must have weighed about 175 pounds. I kept going to Caraceni for several years. It was early in the 1980s, the Monte Carlo years, those strange years when I had to wear a dinner jacket almost every evening. I had tons of their clothes because I have a slight tendency to overorder. It is the only time, to my knowledge, that I had shirts made by Battestoni in different materials from those used by Hilditch & Key. They were less classic, made from a gossamer-thin lawn, with superb pastel-colored stripes. I still have some of them. My friend Jacques de Bascher also used to go to Caraceni. He was stunningly elegant, completely decadent, with a very classic look. I wasn't as classic. I was almost forty and I adopted a slightly more serious look. I didn't want to look ridiculous. So I stopped going to the beach and I put on a bit of weight. There is nothing worse than looking longingly at clothes that you would like to wear but that are definitely too tight for you. After joining Chanel in 1983 I said to myself, "You should really go on a diet." I lost something like 30 pounds and was able to wear what I wanted.

IS: What type of diet was that?

KL: More or less the same as the one I just did but less severe. There were no homeopathic products and trace elements on the market at that time. The skin-firming creams, which I used this time, hadn't even been invented. We are really lucky today. Some of the tests that enable you to check your physical fitness were not yet even in existence. But the principles of the diet were the same and it was sufficiently well targeted for me to lose my extra pounds. But I didn't stick with it—170 or 180 wasn't bad for a height of five foot eleven.

IS: How long did you follow that diet?

KL: Four or five months, I think. It worked very well. As far as clothes were concerned it was perfect. Everything looked just right again. Then, when my friend Jacques fell ill, I started to lose interest in my appearance, because I knew what was going to happen. I lost all interest in myself and trivial matters. I felt old-fashioned in my proper made-to-measure Italian clothes. I started to buy my clothes from Matsuda, Comme des Garçons, and Yohji Yamamoto. I went from small to medium, from medium to large, then to extra large. The cut of those clothes works for large sizes just as well as for small. I wasn't really worried about my weight. It wasn't important to me. Then during the 1990s I let myself go more and more because I was too busy. I had other priorities—collections, fashion houses, photography—I was no longer my main interest. Perhaps my narcissism had disappeared, or was on the back burner, I don't know. And then suddenly, about five years ago, I said to myself: "You ought to take a closer look at yourself, have a makeover." But before changing my image, I made a clean sweep around myself. I sold everything that was linked to my past—because I didn't want my future to be linked to the physical manifestations of my past. I didn't want to be the keeper of my own past, which forced me to invent my future late in the day. It took me three years to get rid of everything then to start in on my weight. I didn't want to enter the new millennium with my old body. I took a completely professional look at things and said to myself, "If you want to go on doing what you do, you need a new look. Times have changed and it is in your best interest to change too before you become a pale imitation of yourself. So stop thinking about it and go on diet. You want to wear the clothes you see but in the state you're in, those clothes just look bad on you."

IS: **It's sort of like the story of Dorian Gray but the other way around.**

KL: I was the picture before, or almost.

IS: **You wanted to change your shape because you liked the one you saw in the men's collections. That's unusual!**

KL: But it's true. Apart from the big shirts, I couldn't find anything exciting in my closet. Some clothes had even become too tight. It's fun to wake up in the morning and to be frivolous enough to wonder what you are going to wear today. Why can't men do that too?

After thinking for six months, I went back to my doctor. Actually, I had to find a new one with the same training because the previous one had died. (He was seventy-six but he only looked sixty.) I met Dr. Houdret and things worked out differently. In 1983 I hadn't gone all the way because I was happy with the result. My clothes fit very well and, for my height and age, I looked good. That time, after losing the first 45 pounds, I was able to wear Caraceni clothes again, which I had kept. I was delighted to be able to wear what I had worn fifteen or twenty years earlier, but the look was outdated. I looked like some imitation of my past. I said to myself: "That's not what you're looking for. You need something different." I wanted something much more striking. At my age I don't need to be a sexy bundle of muscles, thank you very much. I'm at an age when it's better to worry about what you look like dressed rather than undressed. I didn't go on this diet for health reasons. I was in the best of health, thank God. I did it to be able to wear the clothes I saw. That's the beauty of it. So I said to Dr. Houdret: "Let's keep going." I lost some more weight. When I started wearing jeans again, I bought a size 31: I was delighted, I had never expected that to be possible. Now I wear a 26. At the end of my diet, I had lost 92 pounds. I stopped losing weight ten months ago but I am still quite disciplined: you have to eat certain types of foods, give up sugar, cream, rice, eat at certain times of day, and not drink, apart from pints and pints of water, Diet Pepsi, tea in the morning, and espresso after lunch.

Today I prefer ready-to-wear clothes…clothes that were not designed especially for me. I don't know why but Slimane's designs for Dior fit me perfectly. These clothes were designed for young men but they fit me just as if they had been designed for me. Size 46 jackets (because of my shoulder width), size 44 trousers (the smallest French size). I still can hardly believe it.

IS: **I would love to know how much time went by between your deciding to go on a diet and the moment when you really got started.**

KL: Oh, less than three days. I went to the doctor right away but I had to wait about a week for all the test results. Before putting me on a diet he wanted me to have a checkup.

IS: **And what did you eat during the week when you were waiting for the results?**

KL: I ate normally.

IS: **Normally; because you knew that you were going to start?**

KL: No, it was like people who are waiting for the electric chair or the guillotine—they get a good meal beforehand.

IS: **At the beginning, did you find it complicated or excruciating?**

KL: For me a diet without complicated instructions is not a diet. I need discipline to prepare all those little pills, which have to be taken at breakfast, lunch, and dinner. It's just as important to do this or that at lunch as at dinner. The little rituals are essential. If they don't form part of the diet, I don't believe in it. It has to be a sort of punishment, something that you have to do, even if you haven't imposed it on yourself. Quite a while later—after four or five months—I started the skin treatments. At the beginning, the skin is not in danger because there is enough fat under it. After a few months I discussed it with the doctor. I asked him: "Don't you think that it will all fall apart if I lose any more weight?" I was talking about my face but also the rest of me. It has to be said that there are some fantastic skin creams around today. They didn't exist twenty years ago. But you have to use them morning and night. You must never go to bed without cleansing your skin and putting creams on your face and body. Today you have to cleanse your skin as if you had been wearing makeup, just to remove the grime. I remember that when I was twenty-four my mother called to wish me happy birthday and said: "Oh, by the way, from twenty-four onwards it's downhill all the way. So you should really start taking precautions now. You can say goodbye to your youth." I don't know why she chose twenty-four but I have remembered it all my life. I remember exactly which room I was in when she called me.

IS: And you really started taking care of your skin after that?

KL: Yes, but I have to admit that I never gave her credit for it. She didn't have the same criteria as I did, I suppose. She always said things that applied to her, such as: "No short-sleeved dresses after the age of forty; your elbows look too old." I never in my life saw my mother in a short-sleeved dress.

IS: Did your mother ever diet?

KL: No, she never ate. She did go on a diet after my birth, though. She was forty-two and, for eighteen months afterwards, she didn't feel that she was thin enough. From that moment on, I was always held responsible for her weight, whatever it was. But I didn't mind. I hadn't asked for anything. She used to say, jokingly, that I had killed off her youth and beauty. When she died at the age of eighty-two, she was size 38 (an 8 in the U.S.). No, she never had a weight problem. And, although I don't remember seeing her eat, I can well remember her talking about it. I didn't take any notice of what my parents ate. I often didn't have either lunch or dinner with them. And people generally didn't talk about diets at that time. Health wasn't a topic of conversation either. However, my mother and father did smoke a lot and they loved wine and what they called "drinks," meaning cocktails.

IS: Do you remember the first day of your last diet?

KL: I already knew the menus and the supplements, so it wasn't exactly a surprise. Food had improved—the products were better. People are better equipped for diet cooking than they were in 1982 or 1983.

IS: The basic principle is cutting out fat, correct?

KL: Exactly. No fat. At the beginning I had a weekly program to follow. It was fairly complicated. You have to be meticulous and very well organized. I remember that the Sunday night menu was green beans and hard-boiled eggs. That was about all. Sometimes I was allowed a slice of bread (which I still eat), but not always. For six months my breakfast consisted only of two slices of bread with half a grapefruit. After six months I progressed to two slices of bread with a low-fat yogurt, which I still eat and like very much. I used to dislike yogurt; it was a real problem. But I got used to it and now I go to sleep dreaming of the yogurt I am going to have the next morning. So I suppose that's a good thing. And you have to drink a lot—that's what keeps me going.

I drink at least three pints a day. I can have tea or coffee. All that water is intended to clean out the system. But I think the reason I have adapted to it fairly easily is that I have never smoked, never taken drugs, and never drunk much alcohol. In other words, you have to be a real bore like me for the diet to work. When you are that boring, you have to make twice the effort, as far as wit and conversation, in order to compensate.

IS: Will you have to follow this diet for the rest of your life?

KL: Yes, but you never know. You may die tomorrow morning or live for another forty years or more.

IS: **Did you have a calendar telling you how many pounds you had to lose in a certain amount of time?**

KL: No, not a single calendar. I don't have a schedule. The only schedule I follow is that of circumstance and desire.

IS: **After losing all that weight, did you buy new shirts or have them taken in?**

KL: Oh no, no alterations. I have new shirts I designed myself. I liked those wide and very high "officer-style" collars, the sort of thing you definitely can't wear when you have a double chin.

IS: **How often did you go to the doctor?**

KL: At the beginning, every month. Then every other month. Now we keep in touch mostly by phone and fax, but I continue to be vigilant.

IS: **And wasn't it difficult to stick to the diet when you were traveling?**

KL: I tried to travel as little as possible during my diet and especially to avoid long journeys. When you are on a diet, you need to stay at home as much as possible. Breakfast at eight, lunch at one, and dinner at eight. That's very important. And during the diet it's essential not to eat anything between meals. You can have a homeopathic granule if you are very hungry but the secret is eight o'clock, one o'clock, eight o'clock and nothing between eight in the evening and eight in the morning. But you can drink as much as you like. People never drink enough. I lost something like 70 pounds between November and May. Then I spent August in Biarritz and, when I went back to Paris one month before the ready-to-wear collections, I was down to 140. By the time the fashion shows started I had lost another 12 pounds, not by hard work but by iron discipline. And I could wear small sizes again. I had to return to Dior all the clothes they had made for me, so that they could take them in by two sizes. There comes a time when you can't go on altering men's clothes because it ruins the proportions. Then it's better to recut them. After that I decided to buy ready-to-wear. I tried almost every label in existence and came to the conclusion that Dior fit me best—I prefer their style and they suit my bone structure and proportions very well.

IS: And what about exercise? Did the doctor advise you to do weight training?

KL: Yes, but only fifteen minutes three times a week. I have a tendency to get muscular, so I don't overdo it. I live in a huge place with lots of stairs and I'm always on the go. I wonder if I really need to exercise because, when I dance, I feel like I'm made of rubber. My whole body is very supple. As long as that is the case I really don't want to bother too much with weights. Today I feel like my body is like the wind, something that moves easily and doesn't get tired. When I was in school I used to bike, run, and swim and, when I first came to Paris, I was still swimming a lot. When I lost weight I went back to my pre–twenty-year-old shape without doing any exercise. Today it's as if I am made of wood. You can pinch me anywhere but you won't get hold of any flesh. But I didn't go on the diet so that people could grope me or to be sexy. I wanted to be a good clotheshorse. If very loose clothes come back into style, I may put on weight again but, for the moment, I don't want to.

IS: It's fascinating to think that you decided to go on this diet at the precise moment when a new style and shape had come in.

KL: I don't think I would have done it otherwise. That may seem frivolous and not at all politically correct. The problem with political correctness is that it rapidly becomes very boring. It turns into convention, which represents all that is bad in bourgeois aesthetics. If you go on a diet, you may think that, because you have put in all this effort, your love life is going to change. But the flower of youth never comes back even if you lose 88 pounds. As far as I was concerned, I didn't want to change anything. Going on a diet because of clothes is a completely different thing. It's a superficial reason; there's no obligation; nothing in your life depends on it, apart from your wardrobe. If you have a sense of humor, you can make fun of yourself. There's no problem. You have to treat it as an unimportant challenge and that's why you succeed—because it isn't really important. You don't have to lose weight, you want to.

IS: So it's a way of asserting your freedom.

KL: From the moment when you have to go on a diet, or when you think that you have to, you are paralyzed by it, obsessed by it. I only used to weigh myself every two weeks. If you weigh yourself too often, it turns into an obsession. Someone on a diet can occasionally put on a pound. They literally beat themselves up and think that they have lost the battle. But it's not true.

IS: What else would you like to add?

KL: I think you have to be able to laugh at yourself. To follow a diet like that you have to have a sense of humor. Don't take things too seriously; make fun of yourself; admit why you are doing it. It's a physical thing, that's all. There's no point in pretending it's anything else and complicating matters. You have to give yourself orders as if you were a young army recruit. You have to be your own officer and soldier. The general tells the soldier what he wants from him, how he must behave, what he must do. If you remain faithful to your physical and mental self, I think it can work. That's the secret. That's how I approached my diet. You are a general and you have a single soldier in your army. You must give him instructions and he must carry them out. It may annoy him but he has no choice.

IS: I imagine that, in that state of mind, you were never tempted to stop.

KL: Never. For me it was a game and I was determined to win. I never play with the attitude that it wouldn't bother me to lose—I have to win. I know that in sports you either win or lose but in this case, it was only a question of winning. Otherwise there was no point. Dieting is the only game where you win when you lose.

IS: What do they think of your new shape in the world of fashion?

KL: Some people think that I have had liposuction, that I've had surgery, or that I'm sick. They prefer to think that. I have seen people who have had liposuction and I can tell you that it doesn't appeal to me. I hate operations. I'd rather not think about it. I don't want a baby face, nor to look like a trendy young twenty-year-old. I wanted this shape and smooth skin. I don't know why it worked or in what way it helped me, but the result is the fruit of that combination of discipline and sporting attitude. I would never have thought it possible to lose 92 pounds and regain the figure of an eighteen-year-old model.

IS: Do you think it's important in the world of fashion to be as impeccably turned out as you are today? I don't want to use the word power with you, because you are so far above all that.

KL: I hate power. I hate the idea of it and the attitude that it presupposes. I don't want to embody a power that threatens others. For me that's the worst thing in the world. Things should happen naturally. When a man who weighs 88 pounds more than me talks about fashion, he can talk about it and he can be interested in it because he doesn't have to wear those designs. But in the world in which we live, if you are too far removed from your subject, people can legitimately wonder whether you know what you are talking about. They'll say, "He's all talk but what does he look like? What right has he to try to squeeze these poor women into these clothes when he doesn't make any effort himself?" I had to accept the person that I was in order to go on functioning. I also had to reinvent myself in order to inspire the people I work with. I am tired of the "Friday casual look," the "sportswear look." It may suit young people but I'm not sure that it's ideal over thirty-five.

IS: I imagine that people keep on wanting to talk to you about your weight loss.

KL: That's true, most people find it reassuring. But the people who are most put off by it are men my age. They find it difficult to forgive me for having gone back to what I was at eighteen—at least from a distance....

The only people who say to me "you're too thin" are fat or plump men. No thin person has ever said that to me. I am not thin. I am slim, very slim.

Detachment has never been my strong point but I have managed to become completely detached. I have become detached from myself, from my physical self, and from my mind. I don't know if it's a good system but this time I managed to do something I didn't know I was capable of—to disassociate my mind completely from my bodily self. I manipulated my body with my mind, as if it was someone else's. My mind was not concerned with the physical problems of my body.

IS: Do you ever find yourself thinking about certain foods you used to love, such as truffle sandwiches?
KL: No.

IS: I notice that you are smiling. Why?
KL: You see, I used to like the hot dogs and the crêpes from street vendors. The other day I tasted one but I don't like them any more.

IS: So your whole relationship to food has changed?
KL: Yes, that's true. It's like when you loved something thirty years ago. You see it later and you can't figure out why you liked it so much. I like the smell of chocolate but I have never been all that crazy about eating it. I like the smell of chocolate and coffee. That's why there is chocolate in my home. It's not for me to eat, which doesn't mean that you can't help yourself to it. What's more, it fits in well with the color of my house in Biarritz; it is chocolate brown. And then there are the famous "Rocks of Biarritz," and Dodin-Bouffant's chocolate caramels. You can only find them here and I send them all over the world to tempt others.

IS: **That's brilliant to treat chocolate as part of the decor.**

KL: Do you know what I did at the beginning of my diet? I used to place food in my mouth, but then spit it out again. That way I got the taste without the calories. I haven't done that for a long time, but it's a good way to beat frustration. The height of luxury for me is to have an extra slice of toast. It's the most delicious thing in the world.

IS: **I noticed that you had a piece of toast as dessert at dinner.**

KL: Yes, I can do that now that I don't have any more weight to lose. Everything is very straightforward at the moment. I weigh myself every or every other day. As long as I am 132 pounds or a few ounces more, everything is fine. As soon as I go down to 130, I add a little bread, because I don't want to go below 132.

IS: **Was it an amazing feeling to put on your first pair of tight jeans?**

KL: I had forgotten what the fabric felt like, so I can't say that I loved wearing jeans at the beginning. I like softer fabrics, even though I don't often wear them now. But when I do I'm very careful what I wear with them. Wearing jeans can mean, "This guy is trying to look sexy." I don't want to look sexy. It's not that I don't feel young enough any more, it's that it doesn't correspond to what I want to be. In one sense I am ageless. I don't belong to a particular generation. That's something that has saved me. I even see people much older than myself, men of my generation, who are profoundly depressing because they try to make me believe that they are still very successful. I don't care. I'm not interested. It doesn't bother me that I am getting old and wrinkled. I don't want to be young and cute, but there is a certain attitude that I like, which my father still had at the age of ninety. That's not to say that I won't change my mind but, if that does happen, it will mean that the spirit has commanded the flesh to go there. Tight jeans, a white shirt—preferably a dress shirt—and a short, narrow black jacket: this look is associated with me in so many people's minds that I hardly dare show my face outside the house. I almost feel that I am an imitation of myself.

IS: Let's go back to the way you went about your diet.

KL: I put myself on automatic pilot, like a plane. I never doubted the results for a moment, even when they were slow in making themselves evident. The imagination can transform all sorts of personal insanity into elements of self-invention, and you need to make use of this. That's what I want to make my readers understand. Weight is a real problem in today's world. Perhaps it's materialistic but, if you are honest with yourself, you will admit that life isn't only influenced by the mind and powers of reason. It is perfectly reasonable to attach major importance to a person's appearance (especially in the world we live in); the rest is easier to express. It's not only a question of vanity—although vanity can serve as a source of motivation. It is imagination applied to the superficial, used in a creative and productive way. And lastly, it is also a question of self-preservation. It is a lie to think that appearance does not matter in this day. It allows you to live in harmony with yourself. A diet does not need a philosophical explanation, nor all those excuses behind which people often feel the need to take refuge. A diet can help us discover or define our real personality. We are what we used to be—not what we have become. It is often possible to go back, with a new beginning, a different and encouraging one. Being unhappy is not a reason to go on a diet. Put yourself on a diet before you become unhappy with yourself. Don't look to the approval of others for your mental stability. The result of my diet is gratifying, sufficiently gratifying to warrant the journey. It may have been long, but it has taken me to where I wanted to be, where I never dared hope I could return forty years later, without exhaustion or fatigue.

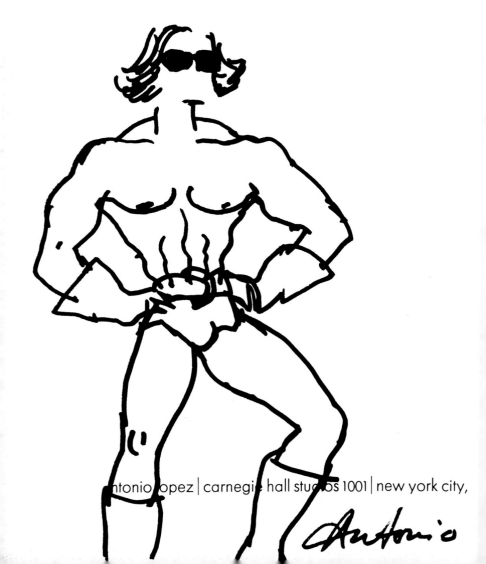

antonio lopez | carnegie hall studios 1001 | new york city,

Antonio

Visual inventory of a person

Photo album

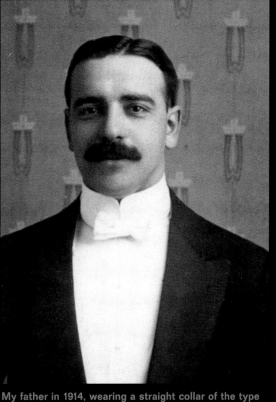

My father in 1914, wearing a straight collar of the type I like. He was 35 at the time.

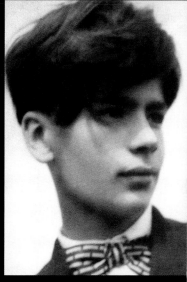

Hamburg, 1948–49. My first black jacket.

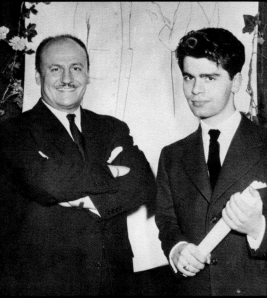

Paris, November 1954, with Pierre Balmain, after I won the coat category from the International Wool Secretariat. I had tried to tame my hair with liberal quantities of Brylcreem. Hair spray had not yet been invented.

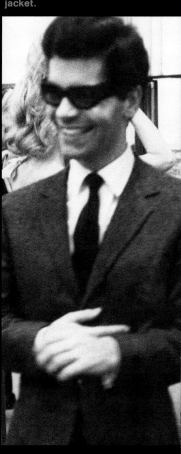

Paris, 1960, at Jean Patou's fashion house, wearing a Caraceni suit.

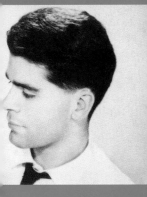

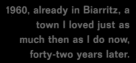
Paris, 1958, with short hair.

1960, already in Biarritz, a town I loved just as much then as I do now, forty-two years later.

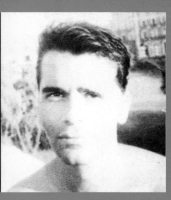

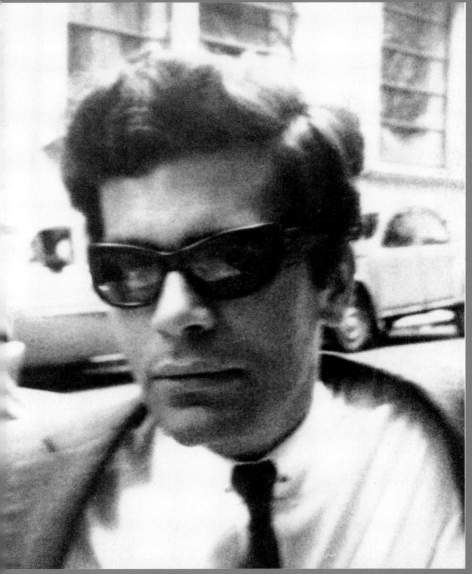
1960. At the time I had a weakness for Ray Charles-style glasses.

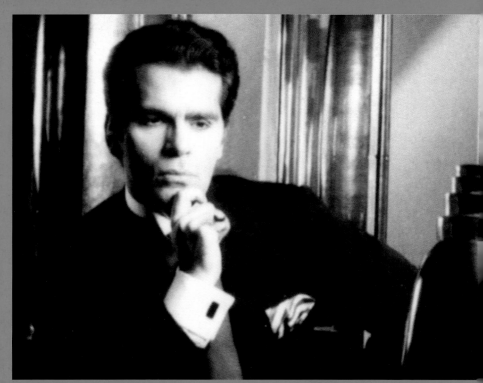

Paris Art Déco (photo by Jean Ramos).

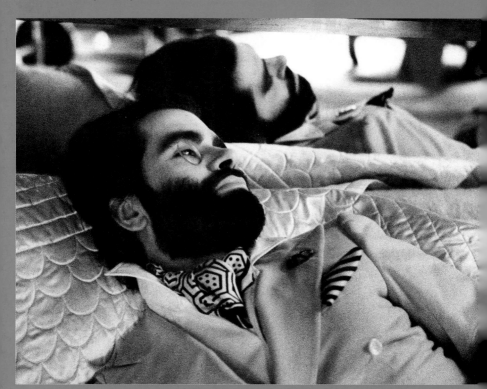

Paris 1973, the "mafia look" (photo by Helmut Newton).

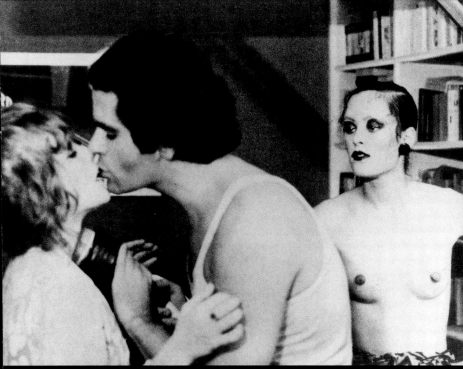

With Patti d'Arbanville and Jane Forth in *L'Amour*, an Andy Warhol film. Is it me? Was it me?

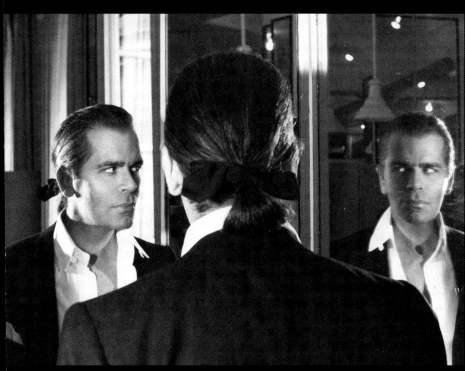

Helmut Newton photo taken at Chanel in 1983. Helmut wanted me without glasses, in an ̣en-necked shirt. And when Helmut wants something....

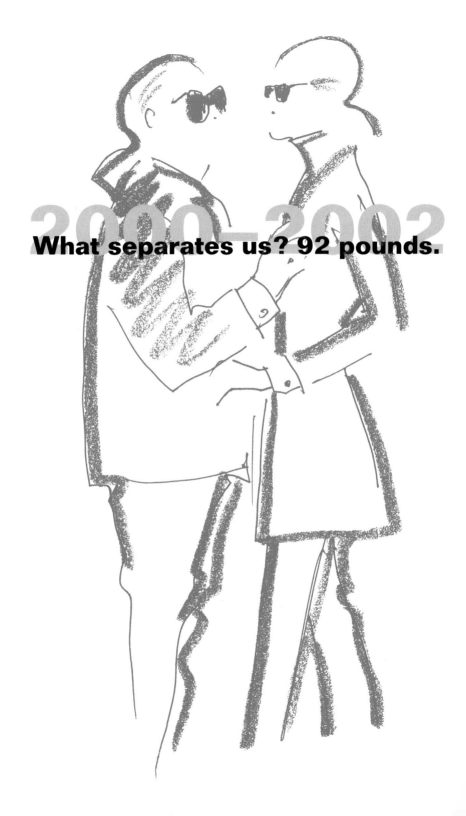

2000–2002

What separates us? 92 pounds.

The Karl
Lagerfeld Diet

My way of losing weight

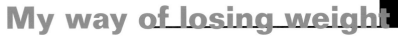

Science without conscience
is just the downfall of the soul
Rabelais, *Pantagruel*

By way of introduction....

...and some figures to illustrate my words....

In order to assess the degree of obesity of a patient, doctors have recourse, among other things, to an index known as the body mass index (BMI), which gives the pounds per square inch of a given individual. For adults, the normal BMI range is more or less between 19 (below which the person is too thin) and 25 (above which the person is too large). The BMI of the current feminine ideal—that of the fashion model—is approximately 17.

Obesity is an ever-growing problem in industrialized countries. In the United States some 50 percent of the population is overweight (with a BMI of over 25). As for true obesity (which corresponds, according to the most common medical definition, to a BMI of over 30), it concerns, to quote but a few figures, roughly one man in ten and one woman in six in northern Europe and more than one man in six and one woman in three in southern Europe. In the United States roughly one man in six and more than one woman in four is obese (with considerable disparities between different communities). This public health problem has a considerable cost, either direct (health care costs) or indirect. For obesity increases the incidence of serious health problems, most significantly cardiovascular problems and diabetes, but also other types of illnesses that are less well known but are not without impact, such as sleep apnea. Psychological consequences, such as low self-esteem and even depression should also be taken into account. The corollary of this weakened physical and mental health is lowered efficiency, even lost work days. Obesity is, therefore, far from without social consequences.

Westerners live longer and longer today, in a world that appears to be more and more permissive, but which is, in fact, more and more demanding. In order to have a place in society, both men and women have to be active, good looking and above all young—and therefore *slim*—even too slim if you take into account the figures mentioned above. Overweight people, who are more and more numerous—for a string of reasons that will be touched upon later on—are paradoxically the unloved of our time. They are rejected, sometimes insulted, discriminated against, and they have more difficulty than others in finding work and their place in society. If they don't end up isolating themselves, they find themselves isolated by others.

Youth, money, slimness, conformity to certain standards of fashion and thought, a seemingly laid-back attitude—these are the pillars on which our society rests at the dawn of the third millennium. How should one accept this situation; how should one play one's game in order to confront existence with all its advantages and disadvantages, and live life to the full without going so far as to obey all the dictates of appearance? In short, how does one come to accept oneself (possibly with a certain plumpness that has gone out of style) without becoming caught up in the cult of youth at any price or using a thin figure to help one along life's way?

In order to live a long and happy life, it is certainly essential to stay in good health. Taking care of one's skin, possibly having cosmetic surgery or hormone treatment, and keeping an eye on one's weight; losing some if necessary. Today's medical and surgical treatments have more than proved themselves. But without the *willpower*, without *awareness*, all the techniques, however sophisticated, will only produce a mediocre and, most importantly, a temporary result. Maintaining or regaining a satisfactory appearance, weight, and body requires energy about one's relationships with others, one's own body, one's personal method of managing stress, frustrations, pleasures, desires…and being prepared to change, sometimes profoundly.

We are certainly not all equal in terms of our propensity to put on weight. But, where losing weight is concerned, whatever your personal or family history may be, the key to success lies in this awareness and willpower. I can help you to lose weight, of course; my method and the Spoonlight weight loss program, which is derived from it, have been devised to help and support you in this self-conquest. But without active participation on your part, there's no point in expecting any lasting result.

Do not begin my program to please your spouse or family or because you have been forced to. Begin it because you want to. Only then will it be able to help you on your way....

Jean-Claude Houdret

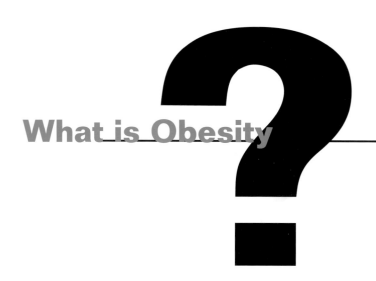

What is Obesity **?**

The medical definition of obesity

According to the World Health Organization (WHO), obesity is an "excess of fat, having harmful consequences for health." This excess of fatty tissue may be spread all over the body, but is generally predominant:

- on the thighs, stomach, pelvis, and breasts (known as gynoid obesity and normally affecting women);
- on the stomach, back, shoulders, and neck (known as android obesity and normally affecting men);
- or inside the abdomen, around the intestines (known as visceral obesity).

Gynoid obesity, however unappealing it may look, carries few health risks. Android and visceral obesity, however, do increase the risk of cardiovascular disease, hypertension, and stress.

In the medical sense of the term, obesity is well and truly an illness. From the societal point of view, it's another matter entirely....

Medical obesity or social obesity?

The very notion of obesity is often subjective because it can depend on the image that someone has of his or her own body. One person will feel fine at a certain weight for a certain height, whereas another who weighs exactly the same and is the same height will consider himself obese and will not rest until he has lost the extra pounds.

The aesthetic criteria of fashion are often factors in the judgements that people make of how they look. Comparisons with examples seen in the media are also a determining factor. People want to look as much as possible like the shape that's in style, and it so happens that, for about fifty years, the shape has been slim, even thin. In addition, many people, especially women, judge themselves (or are judged by their families) to be too fat even when a doctor would say that they are of normal weight. Conversely, many Western women would be considered (much) too thin in other parts of the world, even though Western examples of perfection have begun to spread via advertising and television.

Even the medical profession has been affected by trends in its attempt to define the ideal weight. Thus, the recommended weight for women for North America has fallen considerably since the Second World War, whereas the ideal weight for men has stayed practically the same.

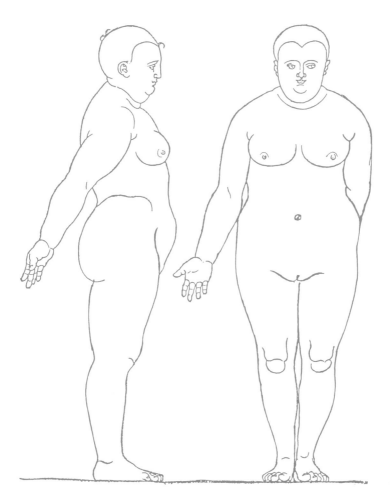

Are you too fat?

In order to diagnose the extent of someone's obesity, doctors have recourse to several methods, the most common being the body mass index (BMI), which I mentioned in my introduction. The calculation involves dividing the weight in pounds by the square of the height in inches, and multiplying the result by 703.

Example: BMI calculation for a woman who weighs 150 pounds and is five foot five: BMI = $(150 \div 65^2) \times 703 = 25$

- A healthy BMI is between 19 and 25.
- Between 25 and 30 is considered overweight.
- Between 30 and 40 is considered severely obese.
- Over 40 is considered morbidly obese.

There are other parameters to take into account when assessing the degree of obesity. For instance, a person with large bones will weigh more than one with small bones, without being too fat. You can get a good idea of bone size from the circumference of the wrist or ankle because big joints go with heavy bones and small joints with light bones. When in doubt, you can't go wrong by taking the middle course.

Doctors can also have recourse to other techniques to refine a diagnosis, notably the waist/hip ratio, the measurement of the thickness of a fold of skin, and most of all the measurement of impedance (resistance to an electric current), a technique that I use and that makes it possible, with the help of a special piece of equipment, to measure the percentage of fat. Some bathroom scales now come with a mechanism to calculate body fat percentage.

The recommendations are as follows:

- Men: 10 to 19%
- Women: 20 to 29%

To review, as a general rule, a good weight is somewhere around the ideal weight mentioned in the table at the end of this book (pp.217–218). But in reality the right weight is the one you feel good at, and it doesn't matter if it is a few pounds more than the recommended weight! However, it is important that excess weight not cause any medical problems. If it does, it is better to follow your doctor's orders if he recommends a diet.

Where children are concerned

There are specific problems in defining obesity in children. The physiological variations in adiposity during growth periods make it impossible to define one standard. In addition, there is a lack of sufficient prospective epidemiological data to pinpoint long-term risks linked to excess weight in childhood.

The committee of experts at the World Health Organization recommends the use of age-specific body mass index curves for each population. With the current state of knowledge, obesity can be defined as being above the ninety-seventh percentile on the distribution of the body mass index of an age group.

Drawings by Doctor Jean-Claude Houdret, in the style of Albrecht Dürer.

The constitution of obesity:
No two people are the same!

There are two phases in the development of obesity:

- A dynamic phase, during which obesity sets in due to positive energy intake (more calories taken in than used up). You can distinguish between early-onset obesity, beginning in childhood (often very early childhood), and adult-onset obesity (usually occurring before the age of forty-five). The duration of this phase varies from one person to another and can last from a few months to several years.
- A static phase in which the obese person maintains their weight by not reducing their daily energy intake. During this phase energy intake is even (the same number of calories taken in as used up). Subsequently, unless the condition is treated, it tends to worsen over the years.

The causes of obesity are many and varied and tend to differ from one person to another.

Imbalanced energy intake and expenditure

To begin with, it is obviously possible to become obese by eating too much and absorbing too many calories for your body's needs. In this case the calories are stored as fat in fatty or adipocyte cells, which act just like sponges (expanding when weight is put on and contracting when weight is lost). There is also a qualitative element to what is eaten: overconsumption of simple sugars results in these sugars being stored as fat unless they are used up immediately.

The body has three methods of energy expenditure:

- Basic metabolism, meaning that which is needed for the body to function, particularly to keep its lean body mass (the muscles) in working order: 70 percent of energy expenditure.
- Physical activity: 20 percent of energy expenditure (with considerable variations according to whether one is a sedentary person or engages in a considerable amount of physical activity every day, such as builders).
- Digesting, assimilating, and storing food (thermogenesis): 10 percent of energy expenditure (which means that skipping meals is not the solution).

The conclusions we can draw from this will clarify issues and absolve from blame many of those who have tried in vain to lose weight:

- Where basic energy expenditure is concerned, an obese person has more lean mass than a slim one and might therefore eat more, just in order to maintain lean mass, without continuing to put on weight.
- Where physical activity is concerned, an obese person uses up more calories because of the greater physical effort required just to move about. The same activity therefore causes a fat person to lose proportionately more weight than a thin one.

This summarizes all the difficulties there may be in ensuring long-term weight loss.

Carbohydrates, lipids, and proteins

Our bodies derive energy from the oxidation of three organic energy-giving nutrients, all of which are essential for the maintenance of good health: carbohydrates, lipids (or fats), and protein. Energy is supplied by the combustion of carbon, which is derived from food and in particular from sugar, which is synthesized with water thanks to the supply of oxygen from the lungs. The unit of energy contained in these food items or expended by the body is a calorie.

Carbohydrates

One gram of carbohydrate supplies four calories. Carbohydrates are the energy source par excellence, turning more or less rapidly into glucose as they are digested: during meals glucose is stored in the liver in the form of glycogen; between meals the liver progressively releases its reserves. A large part of the glucose circulating in the form of glycogen enters the adipose cells—where it is transformed into fat—and the muscles, which store it for future use as needed. Only a fraction of the glucose enters the cells immediately to be oxidized into carbon dioxide and water to fulfill the body's energy requirements.

There are two categories of carbohydrates: simple carbohydrates, which are rapidly absorbed (glucose in honey, fructose in fruit, galactose, sucrose, lactose, and maltose); and complex carbohydrates or complex sugars (so called because they have to be split into simple sugars before they can be absorbed).

Simple sugars provide an instantly available source of energy but contain no minerals or vitamins, supplying only calories. These consist essentially of sugar and everything that contains it: soft drinks, desserts, etc. They cause weight gain by stimulating the secretion of insulin, a hormone produced in the pancreas and necessary for the formation of glycogen in the liver and muscles. Without it fat cannot be synthesized by glucose. Insulin also enables amino acids to enter the cells and stimulates the synthesis of proteins in this way.

Sugars termed "complex" (found in rice, semolina, grains, potatoes, pasta, and bread) provide a less immediately available source of energy, but also supply protein and contain less easily digestible carbohydrates, such as cellulose, which aids in digestion. Certain fibers (notably those in carrots and oat bran and the pectin in apples) also assist in the removal of cholesterol and therefore help protect against cardiovascular disease.

Fats

One gram of fat provides nine calories. There are two distinct categories: saturated fats (derived from animal products) and unsaturated fats (derived from vegetable or fish products).

Fats help to combat the effects of cold and are involved in various chemical reactions. They are found in butter and oil, and most foods as well: red meat, egg yolks, etc.

Ninety-eight percent of edible fats are triglycerides, of which there are several types (the most easily digestible being those that are water-soluble). As for cholesterol, it is an organic body of fat, present in every cell of the body, and connected to sexual hormones, cortisone, and bile salts. It is synthesized by the liver and therefore does not need to be consumed.

Proteins

One gram of protein provides 4 calories. Proteins are made from amino acids combined in different ways (there are therefore all sorts of different proteins). The main sources of protein are meat and fish.

Certain amino acids are essential for the preservation of life because they assist in the burning up of nutrients, particularly in the liver. These are the essential amino acids (lysine, phenylalanine, threonine).

Hereditary factors

You can be too fat simply because your parents were. This genetic predisposition means that, with the same calorie intake, some people will put on weight while others will maintain a stable weight.[1] However, this hereditary factor is not the only reason for weight gain—obesity is not purely a genetic disease. There is an interaction between the genes and environmental factors, such as dietary habits, which are frequently excessive in obese families.

Genes with a predisposition to obesity are fairly common in the West, as a result of natural selection that ensured the survival of individuals able to store fat and withstand frequent famine. This factor, which used to be an advantage, has become a handicap over the last few decades.

An unbalanced diet in childhood

One can become obese as a result of an unbalanced diet in childhood, involving an excess of calories and often too much sugar. It is, indeed, during childhood and adolescence that fatty cells have the power to multiply—a power that they lose later on. When overfed, the cells multiply excessively, leading to a lifelong abnormality in the number of adipocytes. Someone who overate as a child will have a greater tendency to put on weight because of the excessive number of adipocytes built up during childhood.

The trigger factors

Certain life events may trigger obesity in people who are predisposed to it.

- Stress—whether caused by a serious change in someone's way of life (bereavement, divorce, unemployment, moving away from friends and family, etc.), physical trauma (accident or operation), or frustration (disappointing personal or professional circumstances, boredom, etc.)—frequently provokes a change in dietary habits, such as binge eating or excessive snacking between meals. The daily calorie intake then becomes greater than required, and reserves of fat are built up. It is as if the part of the brain controlling the "thermostat" of weight and appetite ceases to function under the effect of stress.

- It is not uncommon to see an elderly woman, recently widowed, put on 10 pounds or more in a few months (despite having gone through menopause several years earlier without putting on so much as an ounce) because of compulsive eating in an attempt to drown her sorrows and fill the void in her life. It is equally common to see people become plump after breaking a bone and being temporarily immobilized; in this case there are two reasons for the weight gain: increased snacking and lower calorie expenditure.

- Certain positive changes in lifestyle (marriage, motherhood, social success) are often, despite not being stressful, causes for weight gain. There is a change in the rhythm of life, people exercise less and less because they have less and less time, they settle down, they eat more because they are better off and more regularly because they have a family. Little by little, the daily calorie intake increases and exceeds to an ever greater extent the daily requirement—which is, in itself, lessened because of reduced physical activity.

- There is the classic case—starting to go out of style in urban areas—of "letting yourself go." There is the potbellied man whose wife, after a few years of marriage, has trouble recognizing the slim and dashing Adonis she married! Or the woman who, once her children have been born, feels that it's time to let motherhood supercede romance—to the great displeasure of her partner.

- Giving up exercise often leads to weight gain, sometimes in the extreme, because your calorie requirement goes down while the former athlete continues to eat the same way: when he was burning 4,000 to 5,000 calories per day, he needed large quantities of food. Once the exercise ends, his voracious appetite remains.

- Giving up smoking is a frequent cause of weight gain for three reasons. First, there is the compensatory factor of putting a treat in your mouth instead of a cigarette. Secondly, the consumption of tobacco makes you burn roughly 8 calories per cigarette, or 160 calories per pack. Finally, nicotine acts as an appetite suppressant, so that giving it up gives the appetite free rein. It is therefore wise to keep a close eye on your diet when you give up smoking.

- For women, periods of life when hormones are changing (puberty, pregnancy, and menopause) are often times when considerable weight is gained. Not all women are affected, though, since heredity plays an important part in the onset of this type of obesity.

The appetite, a cerebral matter

It is thanks to our brain that we know whether we are hungry or full. The areas controlling appetite are found in the hypothalamus, and the neurotransmitters responsible for sending "information" to these areas are dopamine, serotonin, adrenaline, and noradrenaline. This explains the effect of amphetamines, which can radically reduce appetite: they increase the flow of dopamine and adrenaline from the area controlling hunger, thus acting as appetite suppressants.

Socioeconomic factors

In Western countries, the incidence of obesity is in inverse proportion to income level: as a general rule the poor are fatter than the rich. The reasons for this lie in their different eating habits. The most deprived members of the community eat the diet highest in fat. In a world where many consumer goods are beyond the means of those on modest incomes, healthy food no longer is. "Having a good time" when you are poor is more likely to mean eating and drinking to excess rather than taking part in a sport that requires expensive equipment. In addition, the cheap food available in supermarkets is not necessarily ideal from a dietary point of view. The rich also have more time and money to spend on taking care of themselves, keeping an eye on their appearance, and on "self-maintenance."

The main culprit in the obesity upsurge is the modern way of life, characterized by a decrease in physical activity (fewer staircases to climb or miles to be covered on foot), the proliferation of outlets offering fast food that violates the most basic dietary rules, extremely calorific soft drinks, and the growing habit of snacking throughout the day.

Harmful spare tires

Weight gain (following pregnancy, medical treatment, or a difficult period, resulting in eating throughout the day in order to compensate for misery or boredom) can often happen without people realizing it. It is not uncommon to meet people carrying quite a bit of excess weight (45 pounds or so) that actually took many years to build up. In the beginning, the difference between consumption and expenditure of calories may have been minimal, perhaps a few cookies or four fewer floors to climb each day. Then the excess weight began to grow progressively, the increase in calorie intake growing with the increase in lean mass.

Knowing that the ideal daily calorie intake for a sedentary adult is only about 1,800 to 2,000, and taking into account all the temptations a Westerner has to resist in terms of food, it is not difficult to understand why so many of our contemporaries are on the road to obesity....

How I put on weight

When I was a child I was as slim as any small boy from northern Germany. At home we had a substantial German breakfast—cheese, sausage, ham, bread, butter, and jam, washed down with tea, coffee, or hot chocolate, according to how we felt. At lunch we had a light meal, some sort of sandwich that the cook had given us in the morning, which we ate at school or wherever we were. In the evening, very early at about six o'clock, we ate a cold meal that, if my memory serves me well, frequently consisted of herring with different sauces! Never a hot meal.

I didn't really start to put on weight until I was about forty, under the combined influence of dinners out (which I continued to enjoy) and the fact that I had given up bodybuilding. At this point, despite my height of five foot eleven, I started to get round. At first I didn't care; later I began to get annoyed.

K.L.

Docteur Jean-Claude Houdret

PRÉSIDENT FONDATEUR DE L'I.M.F.I.
DIRECTEUR DE MODULE AU COLLÈGE NATIONAL DE MÉDECINE ESTHÉTIQUE
CHARGÉ DE COURS UNIVERSITAIRE À LA FACULTÉ DE MÉDECINE DE PARIS XIII

94, BOULEVARD FLANDRIN 75116 PARIS
TÉL. : 01 47 27 27 33
FAX : 01 47 27 31 08

à insérer p 66

Quand c'est horrible

SPOON LIGHT 1 ***salé ou sucré***
Remplacer 1 repas par 1 ou 2 sachet(s) avec 1/4 l de lait 0% ou d'eau par sachet et 1 fruit ou 1 laitage
ou prendre 1 sachet d'entremet en guise de dessert
Valeur calorique pour 100 g

RÉGIME POUR M. KARL LAGERFELD.
RATION CALORIQUE PAR JOUR : 1000 / 1200 calories

BOISSON : Eau, Jus de tomate, boissons "Light", Pepsi MAX
éventuellement vin rouge *(1 à 2 verres par jour)*

CÉRÉALES :	
~~Pain~~	~~255~~
Pain complet : 3 tranches par jour	
~~Riz~~	~~341~~
~~Biscotte~~	~~362~~
~~Pâtes~~	~~375~~
~~Semoule~~	~~375~~

CORPS GRAS : (allégés)	
Crème	300
Beurre	750
Margarine	752
~~Huile~~	~~900~~

maxi 1 cuillère à soupe / j

LAITAGES : *(Au moins une fois par jour)*	
Lait écrémé 0% - 20%	36
Yaourt	45
~~Lait entier~~	~~68~~
Fromages blancs	120
2 Œufs : 100 g *(pas plus de 4 par semaine)*	160

CRUSTACÉS :	
Coquilles Saint-Jacques	70
Moules	72
Crabe	86
Homard	87
Crevettes	96
Palourdes	168

POISSONS :	
Carrelet	65
Cabillaud	68
Merlan	69
Sole	73
Tanche	75
Dorade	77
Raie	78
Colin	86
Loup *(Bar)*	91
Carpe	104
Perche	112
Saumon	114
Turbot	118
Hareng *(frais)*	120
Maquereau	128
Truite	151
~~Sardine~~	~~174~~
~~Thon~~	~~225~~

PAS FRIT

VIANDES :	
Cheval	110
Foie de veau	137
Jambon *(blanc)*	150
Volailles	150
Lapin	162
Veau	168
~~Mouton~~	~~248~~
~~Bœuf~~	~~250~~
~~Agneau~~	~~280~~
~~Porc~~	~~290~~

LÉGUMES :	
Laitue	18
Endives	22
Tomates	22
Épinards	25
Asperges	26
Choux-fleurs	30
Haricot verts	39
Artichauts	40
Carottes	42
Poireaux	42
Champignons de Paris	43
Choux de Bruxelles	54
Pommes de terre *(cuites à l'eau)*	86
~~Petits pois~~	~~92~~
~~Haricots secs~~	~~330~~
~~Lentilles~~	~~336~~

FROMAGES :	
~~Crème de gruyère~~	~~280~~
~~Camembert~~	~~312~~
~~Hollande *(Mimolette, Gouda etc...)*~~	~~331~~
~~Cantal~~	~~387~~
~~Gruyère~~	~~391~~
~~Roquefort~~	~~405~~

FRUITS FRAIS :	
Melons	31
Framboises	40
Fraises	40
Mandarines	40
Oranges	40
Pamplemousses	43
Abricots	44
Pêches	52
Pommes	52
Ananas	54
Poires	61
~~Prunes~~	~~64~~
~~Cerises~~	~~77~~
~~Figues~~	~~80~~
~~Raisins~~	~~81~~
~~Bananes~~	~~90~~

FRUITS SECS :	
~~Châtaignes~~	~~200~~
~~Pruneaux~~	~~290~~
~~Amandes~~	~~620~~
~~Noisettes~~	~~656~~
~~Noix~~	~~660~~
HUILE "RESTRICAL" *(SANS EXCÈS : CONTIENT DE L'HUILE DE PARAFFINE UN PEU LAXATIVE)*	0

Et, bien sûr, ni chocolat, ni bonbons ni gâteaux etc.

Sucre : ASPARTAM (CANDEREL)

Man should
eat to live,
not live to eat!

As we shall see, there is no shortage of ways to lose weight. I would not be so bold as to say that only the Spoonlight program can guarantee success.

One must also distinguish, to determine the necessity for outside intervention, between being obese and only having a few pounds to lose. Medical supervision is essential for the first group; for the second, a well-planned diet and a little common sense should suffice.

In both cases, as long as the willpower is there—even if losing weight involves considerable personal investment (a statement you can't repeat too often)—losing weight is no big deal!

But once the goal has been reached, maintaining a stable weight, not slowly gaining back pound after pound, eating to live and not living to eat, is necessary: therein lies the problem. The diet is over and, with it, the constant attention devoted to it. A time for silence and soul-searching. Eating badly and eating too much were an attempt to combat stress, boredom, depression, or idleness—or to obey (without necessarily realizing it) the mores of one's social and family environment. Or perhaps one even finds pleasure in overeating rather than in other things. You must take stock once again, make personal choices, radical decisions, perhaps. It is important not to "unlearn" the dietary rules you learned on your weight loss program and to follow a "maintenance" diet. Continued attention to the rules will help you to keep your figure. The changes that you have begun must be made permanent or else the same causes will produce the same effects. As for the remedies to stress, worry, and boredom, I don't have the solution to those. They are the secrets of your soul.

The different techniques

The arsenal of contemporary medicine has three weight loss techniques at its disposal: surgery, drug treatments, and diets. To this we can add the genetic route, promising but still in its infancy, which will no doubt eventually lead to a type of "genetic nutrition" (diets tailored to patients' genetic predisposition) and especially, thanks to better understanding of the causes of obesity, to preventative measures that will be more effective and precisely targeted.

Surgery and medicine alone are not enough to ensure weight loss (and are never presented as such); they can constitute an effective support or complement when used with a diet that is strictly adhered to. Indeed, the Spoonlight method of eating, which I recommend, depends to some extent on the prescription of food supplements containing trace elements and plant extracts. Moreover, it sometimes happens (in exceptional circumstances) that I suggest a surgical treatment, even though the central platform of my method remains the readjustment of a patient's diet.

Let me quickly review the methods, all of which have disadvantages, and some of which, quite frankly, I do not recommend.

The (considerable) limitations of surgery

Weary of a succession of failed diets, many people resort to surgery. As a treatment for obesity, it is indeed beginning to prove its worth, having been practiced for more than thirty years in the United States and enjoying increasing success in Europe. Furthermore, the techniques have improved considerably over the last few years. Still, it's not a miracle cure. Medically speaking, it is used to reduce the risk of cardiovascular disease rather than for weight loss.

If you have fewer than 90 pounds to lose, skip this section! These invasive methods do not concern you and no surgeon worthy of the name would agree to operate on you to help you lose weight.

People whom this chapter does concern must know that resorting to surgery will not cure you of the inappropriate eating habits that caused your obesity. Furthermore, any stomach surgery involves postoperative constraints that the patient must understand and accept *before* the operation (unless he is determined to make the surgery fail and to suffer disagreeable or even serious complications). It is essential to bear in mind that this is a matter of a surgical intervention and not of cosmetic surgery: there is no such thing as a 0 percent risk, whether it be a matter of problems during surgery (phlebitis, embolism, perforation of the stomach, a mortality rate of about 1 per 1,000) or afterwards (complications linked to substances implanted in the body, possibly leading to further operations). It is, therefore, fortunate that such operations are only relevant in a limited number of cases.

Such stomach operations are only carried out on people younger than fifty or sixty, who are suffering from life-threatening obesity, with a body mass index of 40 or above (sometimes lower, between 35 and 40, if the person is suffering from hypertension, diabetes, or any other condition linked to their obesity or aggravated by it), and who have already tried to reduce their weight by a medically supervised diet. A precondition of this procedure is that the person must agree to strictly follow the dietary rules prescribed after the operation and to undergo regular medical checkups for several years.

There are two main types of surgery: techniques known as "restrictive" and those that decrease the amount of food absorbed by the stomach.

Restrictive techniques reduce stomach capacity, so that the person feels full after eating a smaller quantity of food. The techniques have two disadvantages: they cause vomiting and even pain in the early days and, as the body becomes accustomed to the change, they lose their effectiveness. Techniques affecting the absorption of food reduce the absorption of nutrients by "bypassing" the stomach. The long term results are better, but patients are forced to undergo fairly rigorous medical supervision.

- **The gastric ring.** This technique is the least invasive of the surgical techniques, since it is carried out via a laparoscopy and does not disfigure the stomach. It consists of placing an inflatable ring around the upper part of the stomach (an inch or two below the esophagus). If the quantity of food eaten exceeds the size of the upper part of the stomach (above the ring) or if pieces of food too large to pass through the ring are eaten, vomiting or pain (a sensation of a blockage) is induced. The size of the ring, and therefore the amount of food that can be eaten, can be modified at any time by adding to or extracting some of the liquid in the ring, using a device that is placed under the skin for this purpose. The presence of a gastric ring forces the patient, in order to avoid vomiting or pain, to eat less, to eat more slowly, and to chew more thoroughly.

- **Stomach surgery involving clips.** This is quite a serious operation necessitating an incision in the abdomen. The principle is the same as for the gastric ring, but the tightening of the stomach is carried out with the aid of a silicone ring and staples. Its main disadvantage is that it is impossible to regulate afterwards, and side effects include discomfort and vomiting when eating.

- **The gastric bypass.** This operation, which unlike the others is irreversible, consists of closing off the majority of the stomach by creating a small pocket at the top of the stomach and linking this to the small intestine. It reduces the flow of food through the stomach, because food passes directly into the small intestine. After the operation, which is generally carried out via a laparoscopy, the patient quickly feels full after eating even small quantities. Such an operation necessitates considerable changes in eating habits for life.

Medication: use with caution

Unfortunately, as far as I am aware, there is no such thing as a medication that causes you to lose weight, and especially to maintain your weight, without any effort on your part! That does not mean that no substance can have an effect on weight. As you will read further on, I advise people who want to lose weight to take food supplements containing plant extracts known to aid weight loss. As for medications, they are prescribed by certain practitioners to help their patients lose weight but are only of limited value and in no way a substitute for changes in eating habits. Taking medications is never a trivial matter and must always be carried out under medical supervision. Certain "miracle cures" for excess weight are *strictly inadvisable*; these are diuretics, laxatives, thyroid hormones, and amphetamines.

- Diuretics cause loss of water, not fat, expelling mineral salts and lowering blood pressure, thus causing fatigue. They additionally cause a relative increase in uric acid and sugar in the blood by making it more concentrated.

- Laxatives should be avoided for the same reason (too much water loss). Furthermore, they may cause irritation of the intestine. With both diuretics and laxatives, the weight loss is illusory: the number of pounds lost corresponds only to the amount of water removed from the system, with the deficit being made up over the next few hours simply by drinking.

- Thyroid hormones should only be prescribed for patients whose thyroid function is too low. Otherwise, their use causes artificial hyperthyroidism. This does indeed cause weight loss, at least at the beginning, because of an increase in basic metabolism, or the number of calories needed to keep the body functioning. However, it also causes agitation, cardiac problems (palpitations, tachycardia), and diarrhea, then secondary hypothyroidism (insufficient secretion from the thyroid gland in response to the external supply of thyroid hormones). Once the treatment is over, the thyroid gland does not necessarily go back to functioning normally.

- Amphetamines are formidable appetite suppressants with dangerous side effects, leading to addiction, damage to the cardiovascular system, and sometimes to psychiatric problems.

Apart from the remedies specifically prescribed for problems linked to obesity (anticholesterol and blood pressure pills in particular), it is possible to use a medication that inhibits the action of the enzymes responsible for the digestion of fat: orlistat. Its results vary greatly and its undesirable effects are not very appealing (loose or more prolific stools or diarrhea).

The anthology of miracle cures

Revolutionary weight loss methods have flourished these last forty years due to media pressure and the desire to be thin. Unfortunately, the results were often minimal or even dangerous.

Take the Atkins diet, for example, which rests on the simple premise of cutting out all sugar, simple or complex. It is a diet that could be regarded as criminal; deprived of fruit, people who follow it become vitamin deficient. They also face the risk of reaching a record-breaking cholesterol level and developing cardiovascular disease. In addition, they lose as much muscle as fat and will put on weight again, without fail, as soon as they stop the diet.

Another example synonymous with danger and ineffectiveness is the Mayo diet, which has the merit of simplicity but is not recommended for more than a few days unless you want to see your cholesterol level go sky-high and to develop a serious vitamin and calcium deficiency. The diet consists entirely of eggs (four to seven per day). Someone who follows it can rapidly lose 4 to 5 pounds …which will be regained without fail at the end of the diet.

Many other diets have had their moment of glory, such as a certain "businessman's diet," which depended both on a decrease in daily calorie consumption (particularly by a reduction of complex sugars) and on the principle of separation; the consumption of fats and sugars at the same time was forbidden. The attraction of this idea was its ease of application as it allowed you to diet without (really) feeling that you were. But again, the danger lay in the lack of a balanced diet, increasing "bad" cholesterol and the risk of cardiovascular disease.

Other more responsible diets have had their turn, such as the Scarsdale diet, based on the strict weighing of foods for two weeks. A sensible diet, but difficult to follow because of its constraints. Weight Watchers is also worth mentioning. It is based both on a traditional diet developed by competent dietitians and on a system of psychological support provided by group meetings. It is a program that could be described as somewhat backwards, as it reduces its participants to the status of schoolchildren who are awarded "good grades" for good results. There is every possibility that the weight will be regained if they don't learn self-motivation and self-regulation.

I should also mention the strict protein diet, which does not really belong in this list, since it is based on the only principle likely to have lasting results; my own program, the details of which I will give later on, is my own personal version. The strict protein diet starts you off eating only protein and vegetables, then advancing to protein and foods low in carbohydrates and lipids. It is only a good choice when you have a large amount of weight to lose, but it does give satisfactory results. It needs to be carried out under strict medical supervision and carries the risk of severe vitamin and mineral deficiency. And beware of the weight gain once you've given up the protein sachets!

My diets

Before embarking on the Spoonlight program, I had already followed a diet with the late Dr. Richand, who was trained by Professor Ménétrier, the advocate of the use of trace elements. I have always taken trace elements and I feel very well on them. After losing about 33 to 37 pounds twenty years ago, I regained the weight gradually and put it all on again, and even a little more, over a period of ten years. But I must say that I wasn't being at all careful.

K.L.

Balance and willpower

As we just saw, "miracle diets" don't exist. Or rather, they do exist, allowing people to lose weight very quickly…and put it on again as soon as they stop the diet. Worse, the weight is lost from muscle and not from fat. Victims of such diets are therefore very likely to find that they have extra rolls of fat when they start to eat normally again, as reserves of fat will replace of the lost muscle. Most importantly, such diets can lead to nutritional deficiency and high cholesterol.

What else can I say about other methods? My preference is obviously for sensible diets involving a real understanding of one's metabolism and of the dangers of arbitrarily leaving certain things out of your diet and the nutritional deficiency that this can cause.

Whatever diet is followed and however balanced and well supervised it may be, the active participation of the person following it will still be necessary. Losing weight and keeping it off is a question of changing not only your appearance but also your relationship with food; it means understanding why you were eating unhealthy food and too much of it. It means changing your relationship with the world. It is completely impossible to "lose weight stupidly."

My recommended method, even if it does have a name—"The Spoonlight diet"—cannot be summed up by one simple label. It is based also on my personal approach to humans and their weaknesses: a too strict diet doesn't allow enough leeway, leading to failure, stress, and frustration. A too infantile method will be no more successful. Only a well-managed diet involving active participation and awareness on the part of the patient has any real chance of success and lasting results.

My state of mind when I started the Spoonlight program

I started my treatment in the same way you approach religion, with faith and determination but without any qualms. I had made up my mind; I had found the doctor who would guide me. All I had to do was follow his instructions to the letter. I was in a positive and receptive state of mind. I had decided to go on a diet without any particular motive, without any specific medical or emotional problems, simply out of the frivolous desire to dress differently.

I was in the mood for a complete change. Farewell to my magnificent nineteenth-century furniture, which had been auctioned off. Farewell to my Japanese clothes after ten years of faithful service. Farewell to the extra pounds. Hello to modern furniture and minimalist decor. Hello to serenity and dealing calmly with problems.

In truth, the desire to lose weight was just the external sign of an internal evolution. My body needed to be in harmony with a new internal reality.

K.L.

"Little diets"

These preliminary remarks apply to all weight loss, whether we're talking about real obesity or just a few extra pounds. We've all seen it; eccentric methods can lead to weight loss but sometimes to the detriment of one's health and with the certainty of seeing your diet dissolve after a few weeks or even days.

Do you need to consult a doctor every time you want to go on a diet? In my opinion, it is not necessary if you want to lose 10 pounds or less. In such cases medical advice is not essential except in certain cases; it goes without saying that pregnant women or diabetics should not under any circumstances undergo a course of treatment for weight loss without medical supervision.

To lose 10 pounds or less all you need to do is follow the instructions of an intelligent program such as Spoonlight, whose essential principle is readjustment, not privation. This is on the condition, of course, that the measures laid down by the diet are closely followed—no food that is forbidden or not recommended, addition of recommended food supplements (vitamins or trace elements), and sufficient consumption of water. And, it must be said, not playing cat and mouse with yourself, being prepared to rethink the way you eat without becoming frustrated, understanding why you eat badly and/or too much, and realizing that the key to success lies in a fundamental review of your relationship with food.

Before undertaking a diet on your own, start by taking the time to get to know yourself, to work out and understand your behavior when it comes to food. Without changing your normal behavior, write down over the course of a few days everything that you eat, not forgetting what you snack on between meals and dessert, as well as everything that you drink (soft drinks, wine, and other alcohol, sweetened tea or coffee) and work out your daily calorie intake.[2] Also work out your daily water consumption (it is very common to not drink enough). Bear in mind that, except in the case of unusual physical exertion, the normal recommended daily intake is around 2,000 calories for an adult. This will enable you to work out where you stand and to not aim too high; it is better to eat a few hundred calories less than normal for a few weeks than to go on a drastic diet, which could make life unbearable for those around you and for yourself!

Lastly, take a look at the tricky situations that tempt you to eat badly and/or too much and work out ways to avoid them; some people can't resist snacking in front of the television before dinner, others can't resist nibbling with snacks. Anticipate and eliminate these situations as far ahead as possible.

Dieting or cosmetic surgery?

If your BMI is 25 or less, you are not overweight from a medical point of view. If in doubt, consult a dietitian or a doctor who will be able to judge—using the methods outlined above and taking into account your build, sex, and age—whether or not you have a few pounds to lose.

You may, indeed, be a little plump. It's also possible to be quite slim but have isolated fatty deposits, particularly of cellulite. A diet is not recommended for such problems, as you risk ending up with hollow cheeks and endangering your health long before your efforts have any effect on the areas distressing you. What is needed is a specific treatment. Among the numerous treatments for cellulite, the following are worth mentioning:

- Mesotherapy: a method of treatment with injections from several small needles. The disadvantages are that it is relatively painful and has to be repeated at frequent intervals.
- Massage: lymphatic drainage.
- Thermal treatments: thalassotherapy.
- Cosmetic surgery: liposuction, undoubtedly the best method of treatment, on condition that the area to be treated is fairly localized and that the subcutaneous tissues and muscles are in good condition.

Questions and appraisal

Do you have more than 10 pounds to lose and are truly determined to lose the excess weight? The next step is to consult a practitioner trained in the Spoonlight program. This first meeting will consist of a health checkup, absolutely essential to prevent any problems when you are dieting. The doctor will also prescribe you the correct food supplements. You will therefore have to answer a certain number of unsurprising questions of the type asked by any conscientious practitioner before embarking on any kind of treatment.

What is your state of health? What illnesses have you had? Are you on any course of treatment at the moment? Have you followed any other treatment in the past? Do you suffer from circulatory problems, constipation, etc.? Do you suffer from depression or have you in the past? What is your family background? Do certain illnesses such as diabetes or asthma run in your family? Is your menstrual cycle normal? Do you suffer from PMT? If you are going through menopause, when did this start? Do you suffer from any problems linked to menopause, such as hot flushes, insomnia, migraines, etc.?

This "interrogation" will be followed by a clinical examination (listening to your chest, taking your blood pressure, etc.), and of course you will be weighed and your BMI will be calculated. For very overweight people or those with a specific health problem, such as diabetes, a blood test will be necessary in order to work out the correct dosage of cholesterol, triglycerides, minerals, vitamins, magnesium, etc. In such cases the diet will not be able to begin until the results are in (a delay of a few days at the most).

First contact

I first came to see Dr. Houdret because I knew he had taken over from Dr. Richand and that he practiced the same methods, based on trace elements, as those carried out by Professor Ménétrier. Next, I asked Dr. Houdret to explain who he was, what he had done, what he was doing, and how he went about treating people. I listened attentively and then said, "Goodbye, I will go away and think about it." The following week I decided to give Dr. Houdret's diet a try. I went back to see him and together we began on this great enterprise, under his supervision.

K.L.

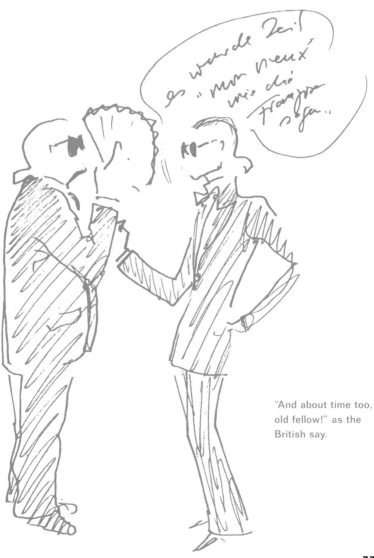

"And about time too, old fellow!" as the British say.

Setting yourself an objective

I may as well remind you right away. However much it may annoy my readers and put them off ever starting a diet, there is no such thing as a miracle diet. And, even if it is possible to lose weight, it is often completely unrealistic to hope to regain the "wasp waist" you had at the age of twenty. Nevertheless, losing some weight, even if it is less than you had hoped, will contribute to making your existence much more pleasant, both in terms of general well-being and the pleasure you will have looking in the mirror.

Many people come into my office and say right away, "Dr. Houdret, I want to lose 20, 30, 40, or 50 pounds." It's up to me to persuade you to set yourself a reasonable objective.

And that's reasonable in more than one sense. First of all, the more overweight someone is, the more difficult it is to get rid of it all. The precise estimation of how overweight you are will therefore be a primary consideration: someone who is severely overweight will have less chance of regaining their former slenderness than someone with only 10 or 20 pounds to lose.

Moreover, the longer you have been overweight, the more difficult it will be to lose weight. When were you last at your ideal weight? If it was more than ten years ago, it will be more difficult than if it was more recently.

Finally and most importantly, are you really ready to go on a diet? Is this the right moment? Do you have enough moral strength? If not, it may be better to simply work on maintaining your current weight and to put off the decision to a more propitious moment. Without real commitment, without the determination to understand and accept the diet, all those who embark upon it are destined to failure.

My objective

My objective was to get to 154 pounds in a year so I would be able to wear different clothes. I wanted to change my look; I had to lose weight to be able to wear tight-fitting clothes. The challenge was to knock off eight sizes to get into my new clothes and feel comfortable in them. Thirteen months later I weighed 132 and I could wear the tightest clothes on the market.

K.L.

Getting to know yourself in order to start off on the right foot

At your first meeting the doctor will question you closely about your dietary habits. Don't be put off by this avalanche of questions. The aim is just to establish your dietary habits and your daily calorie intake and to know to what extent you will be able to adapt them to a diet—two essential points, as you will learn, when it comes to weight loss. The questions will be:

What do you eat and drink in the morning, at lunchtime, and at night, and in what quantities? Do you drink water with your meals? Do you have soft drinks, even diet ones (containing artificial sweeteners)? Alcohol? If so, what (cocktails, beer, wine, digestifs, etc.)? Do you prefer sweet or savory foods? Do you suffer from binge eating? Do you sometimes have cravings? Where do you usually have your lunch and evening meals (at a restaurant, fast food, in the cafeteria, etc.)?

My dietary habits before starting the Spoonlight program

I put on weight gradually, without realizing it, just by eating well and enjoying the things I liked. The splendid breakfasts at the Café Flore, with their sliced gruyère and their inimitable Frankfurter sausages. The wonderful cold meats, the slices of black bread thickly spread with delicious salted butter. And the wonderful pastries, pains au chocolat, croissants, and brioches; the cookies, shortbread, and the famous Kaiserschmarren, a cut-up and sugared pancake with raisins.

Fortunately, I never drank—just as I never smoked. (Let's not even mention drugs.) I think all that has contributed to the fact that my skin has stayed smooth and quite firm.

I am grateful to Coca-Cola and Pepsi-Cola for inventing diet versions. Without these the picture would have been even grimmer... especially as I was addicted to chocolate ice cream. I am speaking in the past tense, as today, fortunately, I am quite indifferent to it.

K.L.

The main principles of the Spoonlight program

In order to help my patients lose weight, I use a mixed protein diet, that is to say based on the principle of added protein.

A person of a satisfactory weight should eat 50 to 60 grams of protein per meal in order to maintain muscle mass. On a weight loss diet, the intake of sugar and fat, following dietary advice, should enable the body to draw upon its own reserves. Proper protein intake, therefore, enables the body to keep the muscles in good condition and to maintain the body's tone and dynamism. In practice, in order to maintain the supply of protein, at least .5 grams per pound of ideal weight per woman and at least .7 grams per pound of ideal weight per man is required.

That is why the Spoonlight program has to be accompanied by protein sachets. I recommend a high-protein preparation made of protein from milk, soy, egg white, and plant extracts with added vitamins.[3]

For those of my readers who want to know exactly what to expect before embarking on the Spoonlight program, the side effects of this type of diet are minor in the vast majority of cases and only rarely necessitate abandoning it (in very rare cases linked to allergic reactions to proteins). They are chiefly:

- Hunger, which may be present for the first two or three days but which generally disappears as long as one follows the diet conscientiously.
- Fatigue, which also disappears after the first few days of the diet unless the instructions are not correctly followed.
- Minor digestive problems—basically constipation, which is relative and linked to lower food intake.
- Feeling cold and nocturnal cramps.

Even more rarely, there may be changes to the menstrual cycle or slight hair loss; these problems are always reversible.

The central principle of my program

My program rests on one central principle: the readjustment of one's diet. This naturally involves a reduction of the daily calorie intake, which is essential for weight loss, but also and most especially it involves giving up red meat. To substitute, I suggest that in addition to the protein sachets my patients eat fish or seafood. This principle can be deviated from in special cases. I allow some of my patients who find this difficult to alternate fish with poultry or even veal.

Food from the sea is rich in trace elements. The most important point, however, is that it enables you to lower the amount of cholesterol generated by external factors. This is because this cholesterol comes from mammals. As we are mammals too, their cholesterol passes directly into our blood, unlike that of fish and birds, which has the opposite effect of lowering our cholesterol.

On this subject, let's remember that scientists have been pointing out the beneficial effects of fish oil on the arteries since the end of the 1980s. The source of this research is the diet of the Inuits, who eat mainly fish and rarely show any signs of hardening of the arteries. Since 1987 many articles have been published in medical journals showing that this theory is well founded. It has since been shown that salmon oil is rich in acids known as essential fatty acids (E.F.A.), notably eicosapentaenoic acid (E.P.A.) and docosahexaenoic acid (D.H.A.). E.P.A. and D.H.A. prevent hardening of the arteries in several ways, particularly through an anti-inflammatory action against plaque on the wall of the arteries and by an antithrombosis effect, which guards against embolisms. In addition, the E.F.A.s reduce the production of "bad cholesterol," which tends to lead to deposits on the artery walls and an increase in the production of "good cholesterol," which in turn protects the walls of the blood vessels. Finally, the E.F.A.s help to reduce the amount of triglycerides in the system.

My second axiom: rather than eating less, concentrate on not eating the same things. I provide my patients with a chart that clearly shows which foods are recommended and which should be avoided or banned completely. *You will find this chart on the poster included with this book.

Furthermore, I recommend not measuring your calorie reduction. What you can eat, you can eat in unlimited quantities. A natural self-regulation automatically comes into play, so there is no point in adding to the stress of my patients by forcing them to weigh everything. This is an overly fussy practice, which runs the risk of discouraging even the most determined.

Three levels of diet

There are three levels of the Spoonlight program, the choice of which depends on the determination and requirements of the patient.

- **Level 1:** A diet consisting totally of protein and certain vegetables (800 to 900 calories per day). I only rarely have recourse to this diet—if the patient himself asks for it out of the desire for an extra-rapid result, even if it means undergoing strict medical supervision. In such cases a range of blood tests and heart checkups are required in addition to a rigorous assessment of how necessary and possible the desired degree of weight loss may be. The patient will also have to agree to undergo regular medical checkups every ten to fifteen days, so as to be able to monitor his general state of health and to detect any possible potassium or mineral salt deficits and to prevent any problems.

The instructions are as follows:

Six protein sachets per day; and at lunch and dinner at least 8 ounces of the following vegetables, either raw or steamed, seasoned with salt and pepper and a little olive and sunflower oil (two tablespoons per day): asparagus, eggplant, Swiss chard, broccoli, celery, mushrooms, endive, white cabbage, Brussels sprouts, cauliflower, cucumber, zucchini, watercress, spinach, fennel, green beans, turnips, sorrel, leeks, peppers, radishes, lettuce, tomato. Drink at least 2½ pints of water a day.

Duration of the diet:

As a general rule, the level 1 diet should not be followed for more than two or three weeks. Only a medical practitioner is in a position to decide whether it can be followed for longer.

- **Level 2:** This diet works in the following way: protein for breakfast, protein for lunch, or the same dinner as for the level 1; the other meal follows the prescriptions of the diet (1,000 to 1,200 calories per day). This is my preferred diet.

  The instructions are as follows:

  Breakfast: tea or coffee (unsweetened or with artificial sweetener), nonfat milk or very low-fat yogurt, 1 protein sachet (hot chocolate, cappuccino, etc.).

  Lunch or dinner: 2 protein sachets and 8 ounces vegetables (as for the level 1 diet).

  Between 10 A.M. and 4 P.M.: tea or coffee (unsweetened or with artificial sweetener), 1 piece of fruit if necessary, 1 protein sachet in the case of cravings.

  The remaining meal: starter (raw vegetables or vegetable soup without potatoes); 8 ounces permitted fish, 8 ounces permitted meat, 5 ounces poultry, or 3 eggs; 8 ounces cooked vegetables; 1 very low-fat yogurt or 4 ounces low-fat fromage frais.

  Duration of the diet:

  The level 2 diet can be followed for several months if necessary (under medical supervision).

- **Level 3:** The patient eats certain foods at each meal and consumes additional protein outside meals (1,200 to 1,600 calories per day).

  The instructions are as follows:

  Breakfast: 1 permitted piece of fruit; coffee or tea (unsweetened or with artificial sweetener); 1 very low-fat yogurt or 4 ounces low-fat fromage frais; 1 or 2 slices whole wheat bread; 1 to 2 teaspoons low-fat butter.

  Between 10 A.M. and 4 P.M.: 1 protein sachet, 1 permitted piece of fruit or 4 ounces low-fat fromage frais.

  Lunch and dinner: starter (vegetables, fish, or seafood), permitted fish or meat (as much as you want) with boiled potatoes, permitted vegetables (as much as you want), 1 very low-fat yogurt, 1 permitted piece of fruit.

Duration of the diet:
The level 3 diet can be followed for several months, until a satisfactory result is obtained.

In all cases (levels 1, 2, or 3) it is important to drink plenty of water, still or sparkling.

Tomato juice is the only fruit juice I recommend during the diet. It is low in calories and is a great help when the situation calls for cocktails or aperitifs while you are trying to follow one of my principal recommendations—no alcohol. Where soft drinks are concerned, only the "light" variety is recommended. These can be drunk in unlimited quantities.

Wine lovers will be pleased to know that they are allowed to drink one or two glasses a day, but take care to drink exclusively red wine, which is an antioxidant and less calorific than white wine.

Food supplements

Dietary readjustment, reduced calorie intake, and protein intake are three of the four pillars of my diet. The fourth is food supplements based on traditional and established plant substances and trace elements. Their role: to help suppress the appetite, combat stress and fatigue, and provide the recommended daily doses of vitamins and trace elements. These essential supplements will provide great support to the patient, both on the physical and the psychological level.

- **A hunger-suppressing dietary supplement**
  To curb the appetite, I recommend, in capsule form, a mixture of plant extracts chosen for their effectiveness in working towards the elimination of waste from the kidneys and intestines: this capsule contains guar gum, orthosiphon, and Isphagul integuments.[4]
  Guar gum (*Cyamopsis tetragonolobus*) is the extract of an annual, herbaceous plant growing in the semi-dessert areas of the Indian peninsula and Pakistan and cultivated in the United States and

Central America. This plant is very rich in galactomannane, a polysaccharide composed of galactose and mannose. It possesses the ability to swell up and form a gel that enables it to create the illusion of feeling full.[5] Orthosiphon (*Orthosiphon stamineus* or Java tea) is a shrub originating from Southeast Asia, whose leaves have diuretic properties (beneficial for the functioning of the gallbladder). Isphagul (*Plantago ovata*) is an annual grown in India and Pakistan. Isphagul teguments bulk up the fecal mass and modify its consistency through the formation of a colloidal, hydrophilic gel; they act together with the guar gum to give a sensation of being full and to keep the intestinal functions regular by providing mechanical bulk.

- **A food supplement that reduces the assimilation of fat and sugar**
  To reduce the assimilation of fat and sugar, I recommend a food supplement consisting of the dried extract of a giant cactus in the ficus family, which grows in the deserts of the southwestern United States and Central America—*Opuntia ficus-indica*.[6] Numerous scientific publications have demonstrated its effect on excess weight and the assimilation of fats and sugars during the course of digestion.[7] The vegetable fiber, mucilage, and enzymes of the plant act on two levels. On the one hand, the indigestible fibers act as intestinal ballast and aid smooth transit through the bowel. In addition, and most importantly, these fibers combine with the fats (cholesterol, triglycerides) and the sugars, and are eliminated with them in the feces. Thus, ¼ teaspoon Opuntia powder "neutralizes" 4¼ teaspoons mayonnaise, 2¼ teaspoons butter, or 1¾ teaspoons olive oil.

- **A food supplement to combat stress**
  To combat stress and fatigue, which are often side effects of a diet, I recommend capsules containing a mixture of ginseng (100 mg) and yarrow (120 mg).[8]
  Ginseng originated in China—where it has been used for some 7,000 years for its medicinal properties. Its active ingredients,

ginsenoisides and adaptogens (which help the body to adapt to stress), are contained in its root. The scientific name of ginseng is *Panax schinseng*; in Greek *panax* means "cure all." Hence the extraordinary reputation of this plant, used traditionally as a restorative and general tonic, a mental tonic (to rebalance the nervous system), a heart tonic, and an antistress and anti-aging agent. As for yarrow (*Achillea millefolium*), a European plant that grows in temperate regions, its active property is chamazulene. It is traditionally used as an antispasmodic, tonic, anti-allergic, and anti-inflammatory agent; its actions complement that of ginseng.

- **A food supplement containing a cocktail of vitamins and mineral salts that provides the entire recommended daily intake**
  Rich in magnesium and calcium, the mixture I recommend guards against any possible deficiencies during the course of the diet.[9] It can also be used for fatigue at any time or as a preventive measure, in winter for example. Each capsule consists of the following:

Vitamin C: 30 mg	**Vitamin B12: 2 micrograms**
Vitamin E: 10.7 mg	**Dicalcic phospate: 120 mg**
Vitamin B3: 9.9 mg	**Magnesium gluconate: 100 mg**
Vitamin B5: 5 mg	**Ferrous gluconate: 40 mg**
Vitamin B6: 1 mg	**Zinc gluconate: 40 mg**
Vitamin B2: 0.8 mg	**Potassium gluconate: 20 mg**
Vitamin B1: 0.7 mg	**Copper gluconate: 10 mg**
Vitamin A: 0.5 mg	**Manganese gluconate: 11 mg**
Vitamin B9: 0.2 mg	**Potassium iodide: 120 micrograms**
Vitamin H: 50 micrograms	**Gelatine: 75 mg**

- **A food supplement that contributes to weight loss helps to balance metabolism and combats fatigue**
  The last food supplement recommended for use with the Spoonlight diet is a capsule consisting of spirulina (70 mg), chromium yeast (10 mg), and lithotamus (200 mg).[10]

Hawaiian spirulina (*Spirulines maxima et platensis*, a blue seaweed from Hawaii) contains over 50 percent protein and numerous B vitamins and trace elements. It helps to fight hunger and contributes various energizing factors.

Chromium yeast is a type of yeast cultivated in a chromium rich medium. It is a cofactor of insulin, a deficit of which can lead to reduced levels of glucose tolerance, weight gain, and the risk of diabetes. Lastly, lithotamus (*Lithotamnium calcareum*) is a small, red limestone seaweed, rich in calcium carbonate, that is easily assimilated by the body and helps to regularize the metabolism. It therefore helps to ensure that metabolism returns to and/or remains in a harmonious state of balance.

My Spoonlight program

I think that I have taken—and continue to take—the full range of vegetable food supplements and trace elements prescribed as part of Dr.. Houdret's diet. I feel very well on them, I am delighted with them, I am neither tired, nor irritable, nor anything at all. I have not undergone any cosmetic surgery, although some people suspect otherwise. If I had, I would not hide the fact, but it has not been necessary. I have never tried to look like a baby or a teenager. I have never felt so fit, so creative—at least that is how it seems to me.

K.L.

And exercise?

It is unreasonable to ask someone on a diet to undergo any specific exercise regime. Firstly because you have to really wear yourself out to burn calories. And secondly because exercise runs the risk of making you hungry. To sum up, a little more walking and taking the stairs instead of the elevator won't do you any harm, but forcing yourself into action won't do you any good. Where physical activity is concerned there is only one rule: do what you feel like.

Incidentally, the activities that burn calories are not always those you would expect. In one hour, someone weighing 155 pounds burns

140 calories painting their living room walls and 130 calories sewing. Why not go shopping (260 calories), play the piano (280 calories), climb the stairs (600 calories—although it is true that one does not often spend a whole hour going up the stairs), walking (330 calories)…or even sleeping (70 calories)?

A little exercise at the gym

I exercise every other day, since I don't have much time, in the room that I have equipped as a home gym. I do so in order to maintain a sense of equilibrium and to keep my muscles toned without becoming overmuscular.

Between the ages of fifteen and twenty, aerobics, swimming, running, skating, and cycling were part of my daily routine. I danced whole nights away. I won competitions in cha-cha-cha, mambo, waltz, and other dances. That's one sport I did take up again.

K.L.

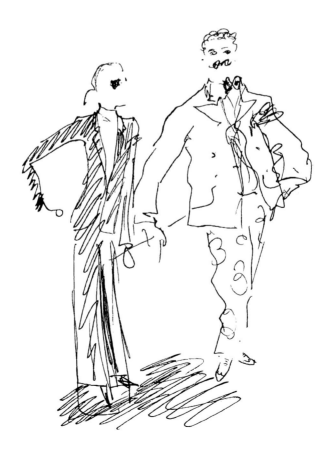

To make the diet bearable

…and to avoid making meals an endurance test, learn to cook and shop again. It would be a lie to say that it is easy to "stick to" a diet for several weeks or months. But choosing good quality ingredients (that are more flavorful), taking the time to (re)discover their color, smell, and look, taking time during the preparation of meals to personalize your own dishes and present them attractively, will all contribute to bringing you back to a style of life you may have given up some time ago—and the disappearance of which may have something to do with your weight gain.

Don't forget that you can flavor your food with all sorts of spices and seasonings that contain no calories at all: curry powder, vanilla, pepper, parsley, rosemary, cinnamon…planning your meals in terms of your diet does not stop you from being creative. Turn to the Recipe section to give yourself some ideas.

Change your approach

- **Shopping**
  Do this on a full stomach and with a shopping list in your hand, taking only the amount of money needed for those items on the list—which will help you to not get carried away—and whenever possible buy fresh produce; if that is not possible, go for frozen food, but avoid all "pre-made meals."

- **Meal times**
  Take your time eating and don't do anything else, such as reading or watching television.
  Put your fork down between each mouthful and chew carefully before swallowing.
  Pause in the middle of the meal and always leave something on your plate (despite what your parents may have taught you).

Only prepare one portion of food at a time, never miss a meal, and don't forget to drink plenty of fluids throughout the day (the ideal is to take in 3 to 4 pints of liquid per day, in the form of water or herbal tea).

- **Cooking methods**
  Frying is forbidden. The following methods are preferable as they need little or no fat, don't destroy the vitamins or trace elements contained in the food, and suit all dishes recommended on the Spoonlight program: steaming (with added flavoring if necessary); microwaving; cooking in a nonstick frying pan; cooking en papillote (wrapped in foil and cooked in the oven); and, of course, grilling, braising, and roasting. The North African method of using an earthenware cooking pot also works well. Whatever method you choose, use Teflon-coated frying pans or woks, in order to cook without added fat.

- **Keeping temptation at arm's length**
  Keep food out of sight and all in the same place. Use the smallest possible dishes and utensils and serve the food directly on plates rather than on serving dishes; if this is not possible, do not leave the dishes on the table.
  Leave the table immediately after the meal.
  Don't keep the leftovers. Throw them away! That way you won't be tempted to finish them.

- **Encouragements**
  Make bargains with yourself ("I undertake to lose 4 pounds every week for a month...to lose between 15 and 20 pounds by two months from now....") and promise yourself some specific reward when you have reached these goals: some little treat or present. Do the same when you surmount other important or difficult hurdles. ("For the first time in two months, I accepted an invitation to a cocktail party and resisted the temptation to stuff myself with

canapés. At last I can get into my suit, which I haven't been able to do for up to three years.")

- **Parties**
  Don't drink any alcohol.
  Decide what you are going to eat that night and have a low-calorie meal before you go. It is easier to resist temptation when you are not hungry!
  Find every possible way of politely refusing food…and don't be discouraged if you have the occasional lapse.

Karl Lagerfeld's summer diet
Here is the diet followed by Karl Lagerfeld after losing the first 20 pounds on diet level 2:

First thing in the morning
1 large glass of water

At breakfast
Unsweetened coffee or tea
1 slice whole wheat bread (1 ounce), thinly spread with low-fat butter
2 very low-fat plain yogurts or 4 ounces low-fat fromage frais

Mid-morning
1 or 2 large glasses of water or unsweetened herbal tea

Lunch or dinner
2 protein sachets[11] (Spoonlight soup, dessert, or custard tart)
8 ounces raw or cooked vegetables and a plain yogurt, piece of fruit, or fromage frais
Drink as much water as you like at the end of the meal

Mid-afternoon
Unsweetened or herbal tea

The remaining meal
For lunch or dinner, according to what suits you best, use the following recipes and drink plenty of water at the end of the meal.

Menu suggestions
Certain dishes are accompanied by numbered sauces, which have to be prepared in a specific way. See the following Suggestions for sauces section for preparation instructions.

Day 1
Baked rabbit spread with fromage frais, plain yogurt, or ½ teaspoon mustard
Steamed fennel with lemon or steamed broccoli with 1 tablespoon low-fat butter
2 plain yogurts, or 1 piece permitted fruit

Day 2
Mixed lettuce leaves, vinaigrette no. 1
Cold roast veal with curry sauce nos.
5 or 7
2 plain yogurts or 1 piece permitted
fruit

Day 3
Steamed cod
Steamed tomatoes and eggplant
2 plain yogurts or 1 piece permitted
fruit

Day 4
Mixed lettuce leaves, vinaigrette no. 1
Herb or mushroom omelet (2 eggs)
2 plain yogurts or 1 piece permitted
fruit

Day 5
Fillet of sole poached with lemon
Braised leeks with vinaigrette no. 1
2 plain yogurts or 1 piece permitted
fruit

Day 6
Salad of chicken breast, lettuce,
tomatoes, cooked green beans,
1 hard-boiled egg, mustard
sauce no. 3
2 plain yogurts or 1 piece permitted
fruit

Day 7
Baked cod with ½ sliced onion, garlic,
parsley, lemon, and 2 black olives
Tomatoes, baked with the fish
2 plain yogurts or 1 piece permitted
fruit

Day 8
2 cooked heads of endive rolled in
half a slice of ham, baked with 3
teaspoons grated gruyère and 1
tablespoon low-fat butter
Lettuce, celery, cucumber, mint sauce
no. 4
2 plain yogurts or 1 piece permitted
fruit

Day 9
Green salad, vinaigrette no. 1
Roast guinea fowl with thinly sliced
turnips
2 plain yogurts or 1 piece permitted
fruit

Day 10
Gratin of steamed broccoli, cream of
tofu sauce no. 6
1 slice cold roast veal
2 plain yogurts or 1 piece permitted
fruit

Day 11
Shredded cabbage, salad dressing
nos. 11 or 12
Tuna roasted on a bed of onions and
tomatoes (cooked over low heat for
30 minutes)
2 plain yogurts or 1 piece permitted
fruit

Day 12
1 bowl of hot soup or gazpacho
(tomato and cucumber)
Vegetables baked in a sauce (finely
sliced zucchini or leeks, 2 beaten
eggs, 1 cup soy milk, salt, pepper, 3
teaspoons grated gruyère, baked for
30 minutes)

2 plain yogurts or 1 piece permitted fruit

Day 13

Salad of bean sprouts, diced tomato, cucumber, corn, celery, vinaigrette no. 1

Veal chop, trimmed of all visible fat and grilled or broiled

Cream of fennel (2 heads of fennel braised then mixed with low-fat crème fraîche, 3 pinches parmesan, and 1 teaspoon chopped chives)

2 plain yogurts or 1 piece permitted fruit

Day 14

Raw vegetables (cauliflower, mushrooms, celery, cucumber), dipped in sauce nos. 2 or 4

Herb omelet (2 eggs)

2 plain yogurts or 1 piece permitted fruit

Suggestions for sauces

No. 1: **Vinaigrette**

1 tbsp wine vinegar (or to taste)

1 tbsp sunflower oil

1 tsp flaked brewers' yeast

1 tsp soy sauce

Pepper

2 pinches sesame seeds (optional)

No. 2: **Basic yogurt sauce**

Plain yogurt

Juice of 1 lemon

Salt, pepper

No. 3: **Mustard sauce**

Add 1 tsp of mustard to sauce no. 2 and mix well

No. 4: **Mint sauce**

Add 1 tbsp chopped mint to sauce no. 2

No. 5: **Curry sauce**

(To go on meat, fish, or vegetables before baking)

2 tsp yogurt or low-fat crème fraîche

Juice of 1 lemon

1 tsp curry powder

Salt, pepper

No. 6: **Cream of tofu**

Crumble 2 oz natural tofu

Add:

1 tsp mustard

1 tsp extra virgin olive oil

Juice of 1 lemon

Mix all together and add enough water to obtain a smooth, creamy consistency

Sprinkle with grated parmesan and spread over cooked meat, fish, or vegetables

No. 7: **Low-fat mayonnaise (1)**

1 hard-boiled egg

1 soy milk yogurt

1 tsp mustard

A little water

Add to taste: chopped gherkins, green olives, or capers

No. 8: **Low-fat mayonnaise (2)**

Add a stiffly beaten egg white to mayonnaise no. 7

No. 9: Salad dressing (1)

1 plain yogurt
Juice of 1 lemon
Flavored vinegar
Salt, pepper, and mixed herbs

No. 10: Salad dressing (2)

½ avocado, mashed
2 tsp plain yogurt
Chopped parsley
½ shallot, chopped
Juice of 1 lemon

No. 11: Salad dressing (3)

1 plain yogurt
1 ounce goat cheese, crumbled
Roquefort, or blue cheese
Curry powder or strong mustard

No. 12: Low-fat sauce (1)

½ tsp mustard
Salt, pepper, and mixed herbs
A few drops lemon juice
½ tsp cider vinegar
2 tsp plain yogurt
A few drops water

No. 13: Low-fat sauce (2)

1 tsp toasted sesame seeds
1 tsp plain yogurt
½ tsp paprika
½ tsp curry powder
Salt, pepper

No. 14: Low-fat sauce (3)

2 tbsp yogurt or low-fat
crème fraîche
1 tbsp chopped parsley
1 tbsp chopped mint
Salt, pepper
A few drops lemon juice

No. 15: Sauce for cooked vegetables

1 cup fresh tomato juice
1 tsp powdered mashed potatoes
1 or 2 chopped shallots
½ bouillon cube
1 tbsp grated parmesan
Gently heat the tomato juice, 1 tbsp water, powdered mashed potatoes, shallots, and bouillon cube. Bring to a boil. Add the cheese, cover, and leave to cook for 2 minutes.

No. 16: Béchamel sauce

Whip a beaten egg yolk into ¼ cup boiling soy milk. Add a few finely sliced mushrooms, salt, pepper, and nutmeg.

Golden rules for maintaining your ideal weight

Your diet is over. The aim now is to not regain your excess pounds.

Obviously, the ideal would be to continue to eat as healthily as possible, using fresh, home-cooked produce, limiting the amount of simple sugars, fatty foods, etc. If you do buy packaged foods, read the labels carefully to determine their proportions of carbohydrates, fats, and proteins…and be careful of so-called "diet" or "light" products. The so-called "light" version of a product (chocolate, for example) contains less sugar than the classic version but more fat and is therefore higher in calories.

Here are some golden rules for stabilizing your weight:

- Take time over breakfast
- Eat fish frequently, meat occasionally
- Never miss a meal
- Chew well, be aware that you are eating
- Don't read or watch television while eating
- Don't eat between meals
- Reduce your alcohol intake (maximum one glass per meal)
- Start your meals with "crudités" (raw vegetables)
- Cut the fat off ham, meat, and poultry
- Avoid soft drinks or lemonade
- Replace sugar with artificial sweetener
- Adopt appropriate cooking methods: steaming for vegetables; poaching, grilling, en papillotte, or microwaving for fish; grilling, cooking on skewers, steaming, or microwaving for meat
- Go back to more natural and less refined foods

*And, most importantly, weigh yourself before breakfast every morning.
If you have put on 1 pound, lose it immediately by going on the level
1 Spoonlight diet for a day or two:* six protein sachets and vegetables.
This is the only way you can hope to keep the weight off.

Don't forget that your fat cells, emptied after the diet, are still there,
eager to plump themselves up again with fat, to regain their former
size and then some. You must be constantly vigilant, ready to thwart
the return of the excess pounds.

By way of an appraisal

I started Dr. Houdret's diet on November 1, 2000, and I think that if I
want to stay as I am, I will have to be careful for the rest of my life. I
don't mind, just so long as I stay slim and fit. In practice, I eat fish every
day, poultry or meat three times a week with vegetables, accompanied
by three protein sachets. In the morning, I eat a slice of whole wheat
bread with 1 ounce salted butter and two yogurts or fromage frais as
dessert at lunch. I rarely eat fruit as I don't like it very much (I only like
pears, apples, raspberries, strawberries, and mangoes), but I take the
vitamins prescribed by Dr. Houdret.

On the outside, I have changed a good deal. On the inside, I'm the
same person overall, just a little improved....

I have held firm, without compromising, and I am happy with the
result. Let's hope it will last.

Dr. Houdret has also given me sound advice on how to keep my
skin looking firm now that the fatty deposits have melted away. After
a certain age that can be a problem.

K.L.

Footnotes

1. Well-known experiments carried out on prisoners tell the story; on a high calorie diet (over 10,000 calories per day) some put on significant amounts of weight, others did not; those who did put on weight had a family history of obesity. (Sims, *Endocrine and Metabolic Effects of Experimental Obesity in Man*, 1973)
2. Get hold of a calorie counter of the most common foods, showing the total calories per ounce (as well as their fat, carbohydrate, and protein content, all of which will be useful if you decide to take your weight in your own hands).
3. Spoonlight preparation 1, savory or sweet, is available in all sorts of flavors—"Breakfast": coffee, cappuccino, cocoa; "Cream soup": chicken, vegetable, asparagus, mushroom, tomato, broccoli, onions, fish soup, pea soup with bacon; "Bread and cakes": bread, chocolate cake, sponge cake; "Omelets": herb, ham and cheese, mushroom; "Egg-based custard": vanilla, chocolate, caramel; "Desserts": vanilla, cappuccino, strawberry, chocolate, orange, berries, apricot, caramel, raspberry yogurt.
4. Spoon-cut capsules. As a general rule the dose is 2 capsules, one at noon and one in the evening, about half an hour before meals.
5. Where the metabolism of carbohydrates is concerned, several experiments conducted on diabetics and non-diabetics have shown that the addition of guar gum to food reduces the incidence of glycemia and of reduced insulin levels after eating.
6. No fat capsules. As a general rule the dose is 3 capsules per day (400 mg each), morning, noon, and evening with meals.
7. Based on work carried out at the Mexican National Institute of Nutrition and by the science faculty at the University of Mexico and experiments made at the clinic for the obese and diabetics at the National Institute of Nutrition.
8. Miltonic capsules. As a general rule the dose is 1 capsule morning, noon, and evening.
9. Vitaspoon capsules. The normal dose is 2 capsules with breakfast.
10. Oligospoon capsules. As a general rule the dose is as follows: 1 capsule morning, noon, and evening with meals.
11. Preparation of Spoonlight 1 protein sachets. Desserts: Pour the powder into a food processor and add 6 to 8 ounces mineral water or nonfat milk. You can mix in a stiffly beaten egg white to give a lighter consistency. Leave in the fridge for about an hour for even better flavor. Soups: Pour the powder into a food processor with hot (but not boiling) mineral water or nonfat milk and serve immediately. The soups can be improved by the addition of small chunks of vegetables (asparagus, eggplant, Swiss chard, broccoli, cardoons, mushrooms, celery, cabbage, cauliflower, zucchini, endive, spinach, fennel, turnips, lettuce, radishes), thickened with thin cooked soy noodles, and seasoned to taste with herbs, celery salt, and spices. Do not add either garlic or fresh onion (which contain sugar).

All the products mentioned here are distributed by:
Laboratoires SUNREX, 12 rue de Presbourg, 75016 Paris;
Tel. 33 01 56 28 14 32; Fax: 33 01 40 67 19 30;
Website: http://www.sunrexparis.com; E-mail: info@sunrexparis.com

Recipes

Whether you are in the middle of your diet, in the consolidation phase, or simply wishing to keep control over your weight, do not forget to make life pleasant for yourself by concocting nice little dishes: for a diet to succeed it is preferable for the three meals of the day to remain pleasant and convivial occasions.

Follow, therefore, the few suggestions here for recipes to help you lose your excess pounds (or to avoid putting them on again) while continuing to smile. They are straightforward recipes, requiring neither particular culinary skill—apart from patience and a meticulous approach in some cases—nor special equipment.

To help you in your choice of recipes, refer to the symbol that precedes each one:

Diet recipe: this recipe fits perfectly into the Spoonlight diet.

Stabilization recipe: if you are in the weight loss phase, this recipe is not yet for you, except in exceptional circumstances. However, it will be quite suitable during the stabilization phase or for anyone who wants to eat well, but not too heavily, without violating the ABCs of dieting.

Recipes for little treats: not to excess; just to keep an eye on your figure without putting your whole family on a diet.

It is important to remember that a diet should never be undertaken without medical supervision in the following cases: pregnant women, elderly people, children under fifteen, people suffering from a chronic condition (heart disease, diabetes, etc.)

Do not forget that the secret to the success of a diet lies as much in the regularity of meals as in the calorie intake: you lose more weight by dividing your daily calorie ration into several small meals than by consuming the same number of calories at one sitting because, once set in motion, the digestive system "burns" the same number of calories after a light meal as after a heavy one. The ideal, therefore, is to eat three times a day without skipping breakfast, to drink plenty of water and to abstain from alcohol.…

Some readers may be surprised by the use of liquid paraffin, which is suggested from time to time. This oil, of mineral origin, is completely neutral, contains zero calories, and is not digested as it travels through the digestive system, resulting in a laxative effect.

Finally, let's remember that there is no point in weighing everything you eat, as long as you are keeping to the rules of the Spoonlight diet and only eating food that is recommended or allowed.

And now, off to your stoves and enjoy your meal!

What to drink!

The best, healthiest, and lowest-calorie drink, the one your body needs, is water. Tap water, mineral water, still or sparkling—all are good. Drink the type of water you like best and drink a lot of it, but don't force yourself; that's ridiculous. If you think you don't drink enough, set times of day when you will make a point of drinking a large glass of water: when you wake up and before each meal, for example.

Other drinks are optional. Alcohol in any form is not recommended; a maximum of two glasses of red wine per day can be included in the diet but I do not recommend white wine or Champagne, as these are higher in calories.

Sweet and carbonated drinks such as Coke and other soft drinks and lemonade are only to be recommended in their diet versions, in which case they can be drunk in unlimited quantities (but be careful of the stimulating effects of the caffeine).

Nonfat or low-fat milk is obviously highly recommended.

Karl Lagerfeld is particularly fond of a ginger-flavored drink, the recipe for which follows:

Ginger drink

Recipe for 10 cups

- 1 cup fresh ginger
- 4 limes, quartered

- 12 mint leaves
- artificial sweetener

Peel and slice the ginger, then crush it with a little water. Leave to steep with the limes and mint leaves in about 12 cups water for 3 hours.

Strain through a sieve into a pitcher, then add the sweetener to taste. Add water to taste. Keep in the fridge with a few mint leaves floating on the top.

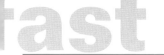

| **Dry Measures** – 1 cup is equal to 8 oz | **125 g** – equal to 4 oz |
| **Liquid Measures** – 1 cup is equal to 8 fl oz | **125 ml** – equal to 4 fl oz |

Breakfast

Summer breakfast
(1 person – 260 calories)
- 1 chopped apple and 4 ounces chopped strawberries, mixed with 1 nonfat yogurt (sweetened if necessary with artificial sweetener)
- 1 slice of whole wheat bread with low-fat butter
- 1 glass of orange juice
- Tea or coffee (sweetened if necessary with artificial sweetener), with or without nonfat milk

Winter breakfast
(1 person – 274 calories)
- 1 fried egg (cooked without added fat in a nonstick pan)
- 1 slice whole wheat bread with low-fat butter
- 1 plain soy yogurt (sweetened if necessary with artificial sweetener)
- 1 glass grapefruit juice
- Tea or coffee (sweetened if necessary with artificial sweetener), with or without nonfat milk.

Breakfast, an essential meal
The first good resolution to take in order to remain slim is to have at least three "regular" meals a day. If you have a tendency to nibble, put together snacks; fruit or dairy products.

Breakfast should be accorded the importance it deserves. It is indispensable in helping to spread the calorie intake over the day. Lunch should not be neglected either, as it helps to fight cravings during the afternoon. Dinner, on the other hand, should be lighter. It is at the end of the day that the body lays up its reserves of fat.

What constitutes a good breakfast?
The essential foods at breakfast are grains (either bread, breakfast cereal,

or toast), which ensure energy in the morning, and dairy products. Items with fat, such as pastries (croissants, muffins, etc.), should be avoided; use as little butter and jam as possible. If you enjoy hot chocolate, make it with nonfat or low-fat milk and a maximum of one tablespoon cocoa. Tea, coffee, or chicory drinks, with a little sugar or artificial sweetener added, are preferable. A final word of warning about savory breakfasts: replace fatty deli meats with low-fat cooked ham or bacon. You can have an egg, but don't have it with deli meat or cheese.

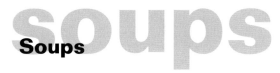

Soups

Lemon soup ⦿
Recipe for 4 (65 calories per serving)
- 4 cups chicken stock
- ¼ cup cooked rice
- 1 egg yolk
- 2 egg whites
- Juice of 1 lemon
- Thyme, to taste
- Salt, pepper

Heat the stock until very hot. Add the rice. In a soup bowl whisk the egg yolk and whites. Add the lemon juice. Pour in the hot stock and stir constantly until ready to serve. Add thyme. Season.

Spring soup ⦂
Recipe for 4 (205 calories per serving)
- 1¼ lb carrots
- 12 oz turnips, peeled
- 12 oz peas
- 10 oz green beans, stems removed
- 2 stalks celery
- 1 onion
- ½ head cauliflower
- 1 bay leaf
- Salt, pepper
- Chopped parsley

Dice the vegetables. Add to 4 cups boiling water. Add the bay leaf. Simmer for about 30 minutes until tender but not overcooked. Season. Serve in a soup bowl and sprinkle with chopped parsley.

Cream of broccoli soup

Recipe for 4 (163 calories per serving)
- One head broccoli, cut into florets
- Juice of 1 lemon
- 1 small onion, chopped
- ¼ cup low-fat butter
- ¼ cup flour, sifted
- 2 cups hot chicken stock
- 1 tsp chopped basil
- 1 tbsp chopped parsley
- 1 bay leaf
- Salt, pepper

Place the broccoli florets in a large bowl of cold water with the lemon juice. Leave for 1 hour then drain and chop. Cook the onion in the butter over medium heat for 7 minutes, stirring from time to time. Add the flour and cook uncovered for 3 minutes over medium heat. Add the remaining ingredients and mix well. Partially cover and cook for 30 minutes over low heat. Purée. Season and serve.

Cream of leek soup

Recipe for 4 (135 calories per serving)
- 1 lb leeks, well rinsed
- 8 oz potatoes
- 1 onion
- 4 cups chicken stock
- 1 clove garlic, chopped
- ½ cup low-fat cream
- ½ cup nonfat milk
- Salt, white pepper
- Chopped parsley

Chop the leeks, potatoes, and onion. Place in a large saucepan with the chicken stock. Add the chopped garlic. Cook for about 10 minutes, then purée. Reheat and add the cream, milk, salt, and pepper. Serve in soup bowls. Sprinkle with chopped parsley.

Cream of endive soup

Recipe for 4 (172 calories per serving)
- 1 lb endives
- 4 oz potatoes
- 1 onion
- 1 clove garlic, chopped
- ½ cup nonfat milk
- ½ cup low-fat cream
- Salt, white pepper

Chop the endives, potatoes, and onion. Place in a large saucepan with 4 cups water. Add the chopped garlic. Cook for about 10 minutes. Purée. Reheat and add the milk, cream, salt, and pepper. Serve in soup bowls.

Cream of mushroom soup ⊙

Recipe for 4 (90 calories per serving)

- 1¼ lb mushrooms
- Juice of 1 lemon
- 1 onion, chopped
- 3 tbsp butter
- 2 tbsp flour
- 1 cup hot chicken stock
- 3 tbsp low-fat cream
- Salt, pepper
- Chopped parsley

Clean the mushrooms. Cut into thin slices and sprinkle with the lemon juice. Sauté with the onion in half the butter until tender. In a large saucepan, melt the remaining butter. Add the flour. Mix well and gradually add 4 cups hot water and the stock. Stir constantly until smooth. Add the cream. Season to taste. Add the mushrooms and onion. Leave to simmer for 5 minutes. Sprinkle with chopped parsley.

Onion soup ⊙

Recipe for 4 (75 calories per serving)

- 2 cups finely chopped onions
- 1 cup beef stock
- Chopped basil
- Salt, pepper
- 2 slices bread
- ⅓ cup shredded gruyère or Swiss cheese

In a large saucepan, sauté the onions in ½ cup stock for a few minutes. Add the rest of the stock and the basil. Cover and leave to simmer for 15 minutes. Season. During this time, toast the bread and cut into pieces. Place a little cheese in the base of 4 ovenproof bowls. Fill with soup. Place the toast on top of the stock. Sprinkle with remaining cheese. Heat in the oven until the cheese is melted and golden. Serve hot.

Gazpacho ⊙

Recipe for 6 (105 calories per serving)

- 3 large tomatoes
- 1 medium cucumber
- 1 green pepper
- 1 clove garlic, chopped
- 12 cups tomato juice
- ½ cup white wine vinegar
- 3 tbsp olive oil
- Juice of 1 lemon
- 1 tbsp mustard
- Tabasco
- Zest of 1 lemon
- 2 cups chopped parsley
- 1 cup chopped chives
- 1 cup chopped chervil

Wash, peel, and chop the tomatoes and cucumber. Wash, seed, and chop the pepper. Place all the vegetables in a salad bowl. Add the chopped garlic, tomato juice, vinegar, oil, lemon juice, mustard, and Tabasco. Mix well. Serve cold. Garnish with the lemon zest and chopped parsley, chives, and chervil.

Fish soup ⊙

Recipe for 4 (100 calories per serving)
*Note: If you can't find fish bones and head, buy prepared fish stock.

- Fish bones and heads
- Prawn heads
- ½ onion, chopped
- 4 carrots, chopped
- 3 stalks celery, chopped
- 3 tomatoes

- 1 bouquet garni
- 10 peppercorns
- 4 cloves
- Pinch cayenne
- 1 cup dry white wine

Put the fish bones and heads, the prawn heads, and the vegetables in a large saucepan. Blanch the tomatoes, peel them, and add to the saucepan. Add the bouquet garni, peppercorns, cloves, cayenne, white wine, and 6 cups water. Bring to a boil and cook for about 30 minutes. Pour through a sieve, retaining the liquid. Purée the contents of the sieve in a food processor with a little of the cooking liquid, to give a smooth consistency. Pour this purée into the soup then strain again to remove the bones. If it is too liquidy, boil for a few more minutes to reduce.

Soup, an ally against excessive eating

Don't feel guilty about the occasional excess eating! It's not a catastrophe, but you are right to want to get on top of things again. Eating healthily also means knowing how to limit excess. Some advice to get you through the dreaded Christmas festivities: limit the amount of food you buy in order to avoid having to spend several days eating up the leftovers. Plan your menus for the week and draw up your shopping list accordingly. Try to stick to it and to do your shopping after meals to avoid temptation. Continue to make at least three regular meals per day, including a generous and well-balanced breakfast and lunch. It is the evening meal which needs to be kept light. The first few evenings, in order to make up for the excesses of the holiday season, you can just have soup or a salad with some whole wheat bread and dairy.

Starters and salads

Eggplant with pink grapefruit ⊙
Recipe for 4 (120 calories per serving)
- 1¼ lb eggplant
- Salt, pepper
- 1 pink grapefruit
- 2 tbsp olive oil

Wash and dry the eggplant. Remove the stems. Cut into ½ inch slices. Arrange on a slanted chopping board. Sprinkle with salt and leave to drain for 20 minutes. Dry carefully. Peel the grapefruit, taking care not to leave any of the bitter white pith. Cut into small cubes. Heat the olive oil in a saucepan. Sauté the eggplant and grapefruit together for about 25 minutes, until golden. Season and serve.

Chicken livers with red peppers ⊙
Recipe for 4 (72 calories per serving)
- 4 oz chicken livers
- ½ cup tomato juice
- 2 onions, chopped
- 1 tbsp chopped chervil
- Thyme, bay leaf, salt, and pepper
- 1 hard-boiled egg
- 4 or more lettuce leaves
- 1 red pepper, sliced
- 1 tomato, sliced

Cook the chicken livers for about an hour in a small saucepan over very low heat with the tomato juice, chopped onions, chervil, thyme, bay leaf, salt, and pepper. Purée in a food processor or mash together with the hard-boiled egg. On each lettuce leaf place a slice of red pepper, a slice of tomato, and some of the liver mixture in a mound. Serve very cold.

Tomato and pear soufflé ⦂
Recipe for 6 (170 calories per serving)
- 2 lb tomatoes
- 1 lb pears (about 3)
- 2 sprigs tarragon, chopped
- 1 tbsp cornstarch
- 3 eggs, separated
- ⅓ cup light margarine

Plunge the tomatoes into boiling water. Remove, cool rapidly, then peel. Remove the seeds, chop tomatoes finely, and place in an earthenware bowl. Peel, quarter, and core the pears. Bring 2 cups water to a boil and cook the pears for 7–8 minutes. Drain, mash with a fork, and add to the bowl. Season, and add tarragon. Mix the cornstarch with 2 tablespoons cold water and add to the mixture. Preheat the oven. Add the egg yolks to the mixture. Mix well with a fork. Beat the egg whites until stiff and fold carefully into the mixture with a spatula. Grease a soufflé dish with the margarine. Pour in the mixture. Bake for 40 minutes.

Tomatoes with tuna

Recipe for 4 (110 calories per serving)

- 4 large tomatoes
- Salt, pepper
- 4 oz tuna in brine
- 2 oz celery, chopped
- 2 hard-boiled eggs
- 1 tbsp chopped mixed herbs
- 1 tbsp mustard
- 16 capers
- 4 large lettuce leaves

Using a pointed knife, cut a round slice off the top of each tomato. Remove the inside carefully. Sprinkle lightly with salt and turn the tomatoes upside down on paper towels to drain for 30 minutes. Mix the tuna, celery, eggs, herbs, and mustard. Season. Stuff the tomatoes and serve garnished with capers on top of the lettuce.

Melon with salmon

Recipe for 4 (90 calories per serving)

- 1 ripe melon
- 8 small slices smoked salmon
- 2 lemons, quartered

Cut the melon into 8 slices. Peel and remove the seeds. Arrange a slice of smoked salmon on each piece. Serve surrounded by lemon quarters.

Well-planned meals

As often as possible, plan your meals as follows: a starter of raw or cooked vegetables (or fruit); a main course of lean meat or the equivalent (fish, poultry with skin removed, or eggs), a carbohydrate (potatoes, pasta, rice, legumes, etc.), and cooked green vegetables; a low-calorie dessert high in vitamins and minerals, such as fruit or a low-fat dairy product.

Tomato salad with prawns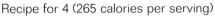
Recipe for 4 (133 calories per serving)
- 2 lb plum tomatoes
- 8 oz prawns, peeled and cooked
- Juice of 1 lemon
- 1 tbsp olive oil
- Salt, pepper

Wash and dry the tomatoes. Cut into quarters, seed, and place in a salad bowl. Add the prawns. Squeeze the lemon; add the juice and the olive oil to the salad bowl. Season. Mix well just before serving.

Raw cauliflower salad
Recipe for 4 (58 calories per serving)
- 1 medium head cauliflower
- ½ bunch watercress
- 1 plain yogurt
- Dijon mustard
- Salt, pepper
- Lemon juice

Wash the cauliflower. Divide into florets and dry thoroughly. Wash and dry the watercress. Mix the yogurt and mustard together. Add salt and pepper. Thin with lemon juice to an appropriate consistency. Put the watercress in the bottom of a deep dish. Place the cauliflower florets on top. Cover with the sauce.

Salade niçoise
Recipe for 4 (265 calories per serving)
- 12 oz canned tuna, drained
- 10 oz green beans, cooked al dente
- 16 lettuce leaves,
  torn into small pieces
- 3 medium tomatoes, diced
- 10 black olives
- 2 large hard-boiled eggs, quartered
- 2 tbsp olive oil
- 2 tbsp liquid paraffin
- Vinegar
- Dijon mustard
- Salt, pepper

In a large salad bowl combine the tuna, beans, lettuce leaves, tomatoes, and olives. Arrange the eggs on top of the mixture and set on one side. In a separate bowl combine the olive oil, liquid paraffin, 2 tablespoons water, vinegar, mustard, salt, and pepper. Whisk well until smooth. Pour the vinaigrette over the salad and serve immediately.

Salmon salad (•)
Recipe for 4 (125 calories per serving)

- 8 oz smoked salmon
- 1 head escarole or endive
- 1 small celery root
- 2 tbsp olive oil
- 2 tbsp liquid paraffin
- Wine vinegar
- Dijon mustard to taste
- Salt, pepper
- 2 tomatoes, chopped
- 2 hard-boiled eggs, grated
- Chopped parsley

Cut the salmon into strips. Wash the escarole and cut into large chunks. Peel, wash, and grate the celery root. Mix together the olive oil, liquid paraffin, vinegar, mustard, salt, pepper, and 2 tablespoons water. Whisk well until smooth. Put the escarole, celery root, and tomatoes in a salad bowl. Arrange the salmon on top. Pour the vinaigrette over. Sprinkle the grated hard-boiled egg and chopped parsley. Serve immediately.

Cucumber and potato salad (•)
Recipe for 4 (117 calories per serving)

- 1 lb potatoes
- 2 lb cucumbers
- 1 plain yogurt
- 2 tbsp olive oil
- 2 tbsp liquid paraffin
- Lemon juice
- Salt, pepper
- Chopped parsley

Cook the potatoes whole in salted water. Leave to cool then slice thinly. Peel the cucumbers and slice thinly. Mix together the yogurt, olive oil, liquid paraffin, 2 tablespoons water, lemon juice, salt, and pepper and whisk until smooth. In a dish, arrange one layer of potatoes then one of cucumber. Add the parsley and the dressing. Leave to marinate for at least 30 minutes.

Chicken salad with mushrooms
Recipe for 4 (60 calories per serving)
- 8 oz chicken
- Salt, pepper
- Lettuce leaves
- 1 tomato
- 8 oz mushrooms
- Lemon juice
- Tarragon vinaigrette (use vinegar and add, if possible, a few fresh sprigs of tarragon and some dried tarragon)
- Chopped parsley

Cut the chicken into strips and brown in a nonstick frying pan without added fat. Add salt and pepper. Wash the lettuce. Seed the tomato and cut into strips. Clean the mushrooms, cut into strips, and drizzle with the lemon juice. On serving plates arrange the lettuce, tomato, mushrooms, and chicken. Pour the tarragon vinaigrette over. Sprinkle with the chopped parsley. Serve immediately while the chicken is still warm.

Raw vegetable antipasti
Choose your favorite vegetables and serve them in small baskets. Here are some suggestions.
- Mushrooms, finely sliced
- Tomatoes
- Zucchini
- Broccoli florets
- Cauliflower florets
- Radishes
- Cucumber, sliced
- Carrot sticks
- Celery sticks
- Green or yellow beans
- Green or red peppers

Serve with a low-fat dipping sauce.

Mushroom salad
Recipe for 2 (87 calories per serving)
- 6 large white mushrooms
- 2 lettuce leaves
- 1 tbsp olive oil
- 1 tbsp white wine vinegar
- 1 tbsp Dijon mustard
- Salt, pepper
- Chopped parsley

Wash and dry the mushrooms. Slice thinly and add to a bowl lined with the lettuce leaves. Combine the olive oil, vinegar, and mustard and mix well.

Season. Pour over the mushrooms. Sprinkle with the parsley.

Stuffed lettuce
Recipe for 4 (108 calories per serving)
- 4 carrots
- 2 stalks celery
- 8 oz white mushrooms
- Lemon juice
- A few sprigs mint
- 5 sprigs parsley
- 12 oz ricotta
- Salt, pepper
- 1 head lettuce

Peel the carrots. Wash and slice the celery and mushrooms. Sprinkle the mushrooms with the lemon juice to prevent discoloration. Chop the mint and parsley. Purée all the ingredients except the lettuce in a food processor to obtain a rough textured paste. Wash and dry the lettuce. Choose some good-sized leaves and place a spoonful of the stuffing on each. Roll up the leaves and arrange in rows on a serving dish.

Cabbage salad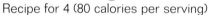
Recipe for 4 (80 calories per serving)
- ½ red cabbage
- ½ white cabbage
- 4 carrots
- 1 onion
- 1 tbsp whole-grain mustard
- Chopped cilantro
- Salt, pepper
- ½ cup plain yogurt
- Chervil

Finely shred the cabbage. Blanch the red cabbage by plunging it into boiling water for 2 minutes then plunging into cold water. Wash, peel, and coarsely grate the carrots. Finely slice the onion. Prepare the sauce by adding the mustard, cilantro, salt, and pepper to the yogurt. Mix all together in a salad bowl and sprinkle with the chervil.

Tabbouleh
Recipe for 4 (205 calories per serving)
- ½ cup bulgur wheat or couscous
- 4 tomatoes
- 1 green pepper
- 2 shallots
- 1 bunch parsley
- Lemon juice
- Salt, pepper
- Olive oil
- 1 head romaine lettuce
- Lemon slices

Soak the bulgur wheat in a little hot water and set aside for 1 hour. Dice the tomatoes and pepper. Finely chop the shallots and the parsley. Drain the bulgur wheat. Mix the tomatoes, pepper, shallots, parsley, and bulgur with the lemon juice, salt, and pepper and drizzle with olive oil. Decorate a serving dish with the lettuce leaves and place the tabbouleh on top. Garnish with lemon slices.

Fish salad with avocado ⊙

Recipe for 6 (171 calories per serving)

- 8 oz cooked salmon
- 8 oz cooked sole
- A few lettuce leaves
- ½ avocado
- 1 tomato
- Juice of 2 lemons
- Chopped tarragon
- 1 tbsp olive oil
- Salt, pepper

Cut the cooked fish into thin strips. Wash and dry the lettuce. Peel the avocado and cut into strips ⅛ inch thick. Dice the tomato. Prepare the vinaigrette with the lemon juice, chopped tarragon, olive oil, salt, and pepper. Decorate the plates with the lettuce leaves. Arrange the strips of fish on top, alternating salmon with sole. Garnish with the avocado strips and the tomato. Pour the vinaigrette over and chill for 15 minutes before serving.

Salads as starters

A few ideas for classic salads to serve as starters: grated carrot (mixed with orange juice), leeks in vinaigrette, mâche, escarole or endive with hazelnut oil (one tablespoon maximum person) and accompanied by apple. Some creative recipes: cabbage mixed with grapefruit, grated raw beet or turnip, mushrooms in yogurt and herb sauce. Avoid avocados, however; half an avocado contains the equivalent of one tablespoon oil.

Chicken pâté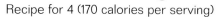
Recipe for 8 (180 calories per person)
- 1¼ lb boned chicken
- 8 oz lean, boned pork
- 4 oz cooked ham
- 1 bay leaf
- 1 onion
- 5 shallots
- Thyme, parsley
- 1 glass cognac
- 2 eggs, lightly beaten
- Salt, pepper

Dice the meat. In a frying pan, seal and brown the chicken, pork, and ham with the bay leaf. Finely chop the onion, shallots, thyme, and parsley. Mix all together and add the glass of cognac and the eggs. Add salt and pepper to taste. Pour the mixture into a terrine dish and cover. Place the terrine in a roasting pan filled with water and bake in a hot oven for about 2 hours. Leave to cool, then turn out onto a chopping board. Cut into thin slices and arrange on a serving dish.

Argentine empanadas
Recipe for 4 (170 calories per serving)

Dough:
- 2 packages (4½ tsp) yeast
- 2½ tbsp butter
- Salt
- 2 cups flour

Filling:
- 4 oz onions
- 1 green pepper
- 12 oz ground veal
- 1 egg plus 1 lightly beaten yolk
- 3 tbsp beef stock concentrate or 1 beef bouillon cube
- 8 oz potatoes, diced
- Salt, pepper

Dough: Mix the yeast to a paste in a little warm water, then add the butter and salt. Pour into a well in the center of the flour. Knead the dough until it doubles in volume. Then roll out and cut into 8 5-inch rounds.
Filling: Finely chop the onions and pepper. Mix with the meat, egg, stock, and diced potatoes. Add salt and pepper. Cover 4 of the rounds with filling and cover with the 4 others. Brush the dough with egg yolk. Bake in a low oven for about 1 hour.

eggs

Eggs

Hidden eggs ⊙
Recipe for 4 (120 calories per serving)
- 8 large tomatoes
- Salt, pepper
- 8 eggs
- 2 cloves garlic, chopped
- Tarragon

Cut off the top of each tomato and remove most of the flesh with a spoon, taking care not to damage them. Season the inside with salt and turn upside down for an hour in order to drain off all the water. Season with pepper. Break 1 egg into each tomato. Season with the chopped garlic and tarragon. Wrap each tomato in foil and bake in a moderate oven for about 20 minutes. Remove the foil and serve very hot.

Low-fat piperade ⊙
Recipe for 4 (205 calories per serving)
- 2 lb tomatoes
- 5 green peppers
- 1 chile
- 2 cloves garlic, chopped
- 4 oz lean cooked ham
- Salt, pepper, and thyme
- 1 bay leaf
- 6 eggs, scrambled

Dice the tomatoes, peppers, and chile. Cook over a low heat for 20 minutes with the garlic, ham, salt, pepper, thyme, and bay leaf. Cover with a tight fitting lid. Just before serving add the scrambled eggs, previously cooked without fat in a bowl over water or in the microwave. Mix all together.

Eggplant omelet ⊙
Recipe for 4 (133 calories per person)
- 2 shallots
- 2 lb eggplant
- Salt, pepper
- 6 eggs
- Chopped mixed herbs

Chop the shallots. Peel and dice the eggplant and brown lightly in a nonstick pan with a little water. After 5 minutes, season with salt and pepper and add the shallots. Cook until all the water has evaporated. Beat the eggs with a fork and add the herbs. Season. Pour over the eggplant. Cook and serve hot.

Omelet with chanterelle mushrooms ⊙

Recipe for 4 (69 calories per serving)

- 10 oz chanterelle mushrooms
- Vinegar
- 1 tbsp butter
- Salt, pepper
- 6 eggs
- Chopped marjoram or oregano

Wash the mushrooms in water to which a little vinegar has been added. Slice and fry in the butter. Season. Beat the eggs with a fork, add the marjoram, pour over the mushrooms and cook in the normal way. Serve immediately.

Baked eggs ⋮

Recipe for 4 (214 calories per serving)

- 1 cup tomato sauce
- 1 lb cooked green beans
- 4 oz cooked ham, diced
- 4 eggs
- 12 spears asparagus
- Chopped parsley
- Croutons

Divide the tomato sauce between 4 individual molds. Add the beans and the diced ham. Bake in the oven until it comes to a boil. Break the eggs over the hot sauce, garnish with the asparagus spears and return to the oven for a moment. Immediately before serving, sprinkle parsley over. Garnish with croutons.

Eggs, useful allies on a diet

Eggs are very low in calories: 1 egg white contains 20 calories with a fat content of 0 percent, and an egg yolk contains 55 calories with a fat content of 5 grams. Eggs have the additional advantage of making you feel full and staving off hunger pangs. They are therefore excellent allies when trying to lose weight as long as they are consumed in moderation.

Baked eggs with watercress ⊙

Recipe for 4 (120 calories per serving)

- 1 bunch watercress
- 1 clove garlic, chopped
- 6 oz low-fat fromage frais or plain yogurt
- Salt, pepper
- 4 eggs
- 1 shallot
- 3 tomatoes
- Chopped basil

Cook the watercress in boiling water for 5 minutes with the chopped garlic. Drain well, then chop and mix with the fromage frais. Season. Divide the mixture between 4 individual dishes then break an egg over the top of each. Place the dishes in a roasting pan full of water and bake in a preheated oven. During this time, prepare the tomato coulis. Chop the shallot and brown in a nonstick frying pan with a little water. Plunge the tomatoes into boiling water, peel, seed, and chop them, then add the flesh to the frying pan with the basil. Cook for 20 minutes over medium heat. Immediately before serving, pour the coulis over the eggs.

Scallops with watercress ⊙

Recipe for 6 (120 calories per serving)

- 1 bunch watercress
- 4 eggs, lightly beaten
- 2 cups milk
- Salt, pepper
- 1½ lb scallops
- 1 cup white wine
- 3 shallots, chopped
- 1 bay leaf
- 2 oz white fish
- 1 egg yolk
- Saffron

Wash the watercress and blanch for 1 minute in boiling water. Purée in a food processor. Mix with the beaten eggs and the milk. Season. Place in individual molds in a roasting pan filled with water and bake for 30 minutes. During this time, season the scallops and cook in a hot nonstick frying pan without added fat. In a separate pan reduce half of the white wine with the shallots then add the rest of the white wine, the bay leaf, and the white fish. Simmer over low heat until the mixture has reduced by half. Purée in a food processor, then add the egg yolk and a little saffron. Strain through a sieve then keep warm, taking care not to let the sauce come to a boil. Turn the molds out onto plates, garnish with scallops, and cover with the sauce.

Fish soufflé ⦂

Recipe for 4 (220 calories per serving)
- 1½ lb white fish
- 1 cup warm nonfat milk
- Juice of 1 lemon
- Chopped marjoram or oregano
- Salt, pepper
- 4 eggs, separated
- 1 tbsp light margarine

Poach the fish for 6–8 minutes. Let cool, then flake. Add the warm milk, lemon juice, and marjoram. Season to taste. Beat the egg whites until stiff and fold very carefully into the sauce. Lightly butter a soufflé dish with the margarine. Pour in the mixture and bake in a medium oven for about 30 minutes until golden and well risen. Serve immediately.

Asparagus soufflé ⦂

Recipe for 4 (240 calories per serving)
- 4 oz chicken liver
- Salt, pepper
- 2 lb asparagus
- 4 eggs, separated
- 2 tbsp flour
- Chopped parsley
- 6 oz low-fat fromage frais or plain yogurt
- 1 tbsp butter

Brown the chicken liver in a nonstick frying pan. Season, then dice. Cook the asparagus in salted, boiling water for about 8 minutes. Drain, cut off and retain the tips, and purée the rest in a food processor. Beat the egg yolks in a large bowl. Season, then add the flour. Add the asparagus purée, chicken livers, asparagus tips, parsley, and fromage frais. Beat the egg whites until stiff and fold very carefully into the mixture. Check the seasoning. Lightly butter a soufflé dish. Pour the mixture into a dish and cook for 20 minutes. Serve immediately.

How many eggs should you eat in a week?

If your cholesterol level is normal, the maximum recommended number of eggs is six per week. For those with high cholesterol the number of eggs eaten should vary according to the extent of the problem. In either case, take care to ensure that the eggs are fresh and don't forget that, although egg yolks are high in cholesterol, the whites can be eaten with impunity. Stiffly beaten egg whites are particularly useful when making soufflés (enabling you, for example, to make a delicious asparagus or mushroom soufflé with Spoonlight protein sachets), meringues, low-fat purées, etc.

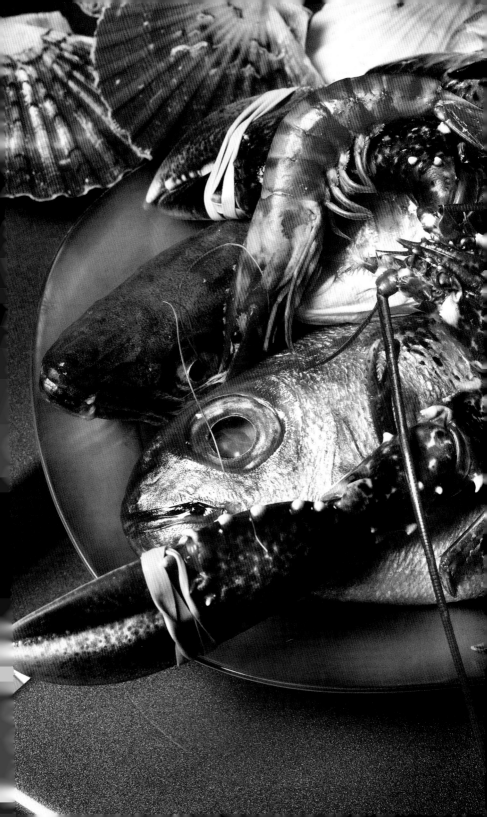

Fish and shellfish

Tuna and blackberry mousse
Recipe for 4 (400 calories per serving)
- 6 oz blackberries
- Salt
- 12 oz fresh tuna
- 1 tbsp oil
- 3 egg whites
- 1 tbsp light margarine

Wash the blackberries carefully and drain well. Season the tuna. Heat the oil in a frying pan and brown the tuna on all sides. Season and purée in a food processor. Preheat the oven to 350°F. Beat the egg whites until stiff. Mix carefully with the tuna. Butter a high-sided oven dish with the margarine. Add a third of the tuna, cover with half of the blackberries, add a second layer of tuna, then the second half of the blackberries, finishing with a third layer of tuna. Smooth the surface with a spoon. Bake for 40 minutes. Remove and cool. When cool, place in the refrigerator for several hours. Turn out and serve in slices approximately ½ inch thick.

Cod with black currants
Recipe for 4 (180 calories per serving)
- 4 cod steaks, about 6 oz each
- 8 oz fresh black currants or blueberries
- 1 onion
- 1 tbsp olive oil
- Salt

Carefully wipe the cod. Rinse and drain the black currants, then remove from the stem. Thinly slice the onion. Heat the oil in a high-sided frying pan and sauté the onion until golden. Add the cod and brown for 5 minutes on one side. Season. Turn the steaks over and season the other side. Add the black currants and cook over low heat for another 5 minutes. Serve on hot plates.

shellfish

Cod with peppers
Recipe for 4 (140 calories per serving)
- 1 lb cod fillet
- 1 onion, thinly sliced
- 1 carrot, sliced ½ inch thick
- 1 clove
- 1 bay leaf
- 2 green peppers, sliced
- 2 red peppers, sliced
- 10 oz tomato sauce
- Rosemary

Cut the cod into even-sized pieces. Place in a saucepan, cover with cold water and add the onion, carrot, clove, and bay leaf. Cook over low heat for 5 minutes. Drain the fish. Brown the peppers in a nonstick frying pan with a little water. Grease an ovenproof baking dish. Pour in the tomato sauce, then add half of the peppers, the pieces of cod, and the rosemary. Cover with the remaining sauce and peppers. Bake for a few minutes in the oven. Serve immediately.

Mussels in white wine
Recipe for 4 (75 calories per serving)
- 2 qt mussels
- 1 onion
- 3 shallots
- 2 cloves garlic
- Parsley
- 1 pinch thyme
- 1 bay leaf
- 1 cup white wine
- Salt, pepper

Clean and wash the mussels thoroughly and place in a large saucepan. Finely chop the onion, shallots, garlic, and parsley and add to the mussels along with the thyme and bay leaf. Pour the white wine over. Cover and cook on high heat for a few moments.

Shake the pan to turn the mussels two or three times. They will be cooked when they have all opened. Place on a serving dish. Reduce the liquid for a few minutes and check the seasoning. Pour over the mussels and serve immediately.

Crayfish in court bouillon

Recipe for 4 (120 calories per serving)

- 3 carrots
- 5 shallots
- 1 onion
- 1¼ cups white wine
- Tarragon
- Thyme
- 1 bay leaf
- Salt, peppercorns
- 2 dozen crayfish

Thinly slice the carrots, shallots, and onion. Steam for a few minutes, then add the wine. Add the tarragon, thyme, bay leaf, salt, and peppercorns. Raise the heat and reduce the liquid by half, then cover the pan and simmer the crayfish in the liquid for 12 minutes.

Monkfish in tomato sauce

Recipe for 4 (145 calories per serving)

- 1½ lb monkfish
- Salt, pepper
- A few slices fennel
- Fresh tomato coulis
  (see page 155)

Cut the monkfish into 8 pieces. Season. Steam for 8 minutes with the fennel. Pour the tomato coulis over and serve hot.

Halibut fillets with mustard

Recipe for 4 (175 calories per serving)

- 4 halibut fillets, 6 oz each
- 2 tbsp flour
- 1 cup fish stock
- 3 tbsp whole-grain mustard
- Salt, pepper
- 3 tbsp crème fraîche
- Chopped parsley

Steam the seasoned halibut fillets for 8–10 minutes. During this time, mix the flour into the fish stock. Boil over low heat for a few minutes, then add the mustard. Season, then add the crème fraîche. Pour a layer of sauce on the serving plates and place the fish on top. Sprinkle with parsley.

Fish stew

Recipe for 4 (280 calories per serving)

- 2 leeks, well rinsed
- 8 oz carrots
- 3 stalks celery
- Salt, pepper
- 1 onion with a clove stuck in it
- Bouquet garni
- 12 oz cod
- 12 oz turbot
- 12 oz monkfish
- Chopped parsley

Slice the leeks, carrots, and celery. Make a stock with water, salt, the onion with a clove stuck in it, and the bouquet garni. When this has come to a boil add the leeks, carrots, and celery. Cook for 25 minutes. Add the fish and leave to cook for 15 minutes over low heat. Drain. Serve the fish with the vegetables and sprinkle with parsley.

Fish: both ally and enemy

Allies: eels, fresh anchovies, anchovies preserved in brine, halibut, fresh or smoked herring, pickled herring, fresh or smoked mackerel, mackerel preserved in white wine, dogfish, fresh sardines, fresh or smoked salmon, fresh tuna, tuna preserved in brine, trout, caviar, lumpfish caviar.

Enemies: anchovies, sardines or tuna preserved in oil, herring in cream, fish coated with breadcrumbs, fried fish, fish cakes.

Prawns in garlic sauce

Recipe for 4 (220 calories per serving)

- 8 cherry tomatoes
- 2 lb medium prawns, shelled
- 3 tbsp vegetable oil
- ½ green pepper, cut into strips
- 1 small onion, thinly sliced
- Chopped parsley
- 1 tbsp marinara sauce
- Chopped dill
- 1 clove garlic, chopped
- Salt, pepper

Pour boiling water over the tomatoes. Leave for 2 or 3 minutes then peel and chop. Rinse the shelled prawns. Place the oil, tomatoes, green pepper, onion, parsley, marinara sauce, dill, and garlic in a large frying pan. Cook over low heat for 2 minutes. Season. Add the prawns and leave to cook for 8 minutes until tender, stirring frequently. Serve immediately.

Fried calamari ⦿

Recipe for 4 (200 calories per serving)

- 2 lb small squid, cleaned
- 10 oz tomatoes
- 1 onion
- 2 cloves garlic, chopped
- Chopped parsley
- Olive oil
- Salt, pepper

Cut the squid into strips. Chop the tomatoes. Thinly slice the onion. Cook the onion, garlic, and some parsley in the oil until the onion is transparent. Add some additional parsley and the rest of the ingredients. Leave to simmer for about 8 minutes. Check frequently as overcooked squid becomes rubbery.

Sole with spinach ⦿

Recipe for 4 (155 calories per serving)

- 10 oz fresh spinach
- 1 small onion, thinly sliced
- 1 clove garlic, chopped
- 4 oz low-fat ricotta
- Chopped parsley
- 4 sole fillets, 6 oz each
- Salt, pepper
- ½ cup dry white wine
- Juice of ½ lemon

Cook the spinach, thinly sliced onion, and garlic. Stir in the ricotta and parsley. Stuff the fillets and fold over at each end. Insert a toothpick to retain the shape. Season. Bake in a hot oven for about 10 minutes, basting frequently with the wine and lemon juice.

Mussels with peppers ⦿

Recipe for 4 (345 calories per serving)

- 2 lb very large mussels
- 12 oz red and yellow peppers
- 3 small white onions
- 2 tbsp olive oil
- 1 small red chile
- 1 tbsp chopped parsley
- Salt, pepper

Scrape the mussels, then wash and trim carefully. Place in a large saucepan over high heat. Cover and leave the mussels to open, turning them from time to time. When they have all opened, remove the pan from the heat and keep warm. Dice the peppers. Chop the onions finely. Pour the oil into a high-sided frying pan, add the peppers and onions and cook for 3 minutes, stirring frequently. Chop the chile and add to the frying pan along with the parsley and season. Mix and remove from the heat. Remove the empty half of each mussel shell. Place the half containing the mussel on a dish large enough to place them all side by side. Cover each mussel with a teaspoon of the pepper mixture. Broil for 5 minutes. Serve hot.

Sea bream with fennel
Recipe for 4 (250 calories per serving)

- 1 onion
- 4 heads fennel
- 1 clove garlic
- ½ cup white wine
- Pepper
- 3 bay leaves
- 3 lb whole sea bream

Thinly slice the onion. Wash the fennel thoroughly and chop. Chop the garlic. Place the vegetables in an ovenproof dish and pour over the white wine and ⅔ cup water. Season with pepper. Add the bay leaves. Cover and place in a hot oven for 20 minutes. Remove from the oven. Place the whole fish on top of the vegetables and cook for 15 minutes longer, basting from time to time. Before serving, remove and discard the skin from the fish then cover with the vegetables.

Summer sea bass with orange
Recipe for 6 (366 calories per serving)

- 1 sea bass, cleaned but not scaled, about 4 lb
- Salt
- 2 oranges
- 4 pinches sesame seeds
- 2 tbsp olive oil

Wipe the sea bass and salt the inside. Preheat the oven to 400ºF. Wash and dry the oranges. Remove the zest from one of them and squeeze both. Sprinkle the grated orange zest and the sesame seeds over the sea bass. Place the sea bass in an ovenproof dish. Drizzle with the oil, broil for 10 minutes, pour the orange juice over, and broil 5 minutes longer.

Monkfish poached in wine ⊙

Recipe for 6 (170 calories per person)

- ¼ onion
- ½ carrot
- 1 cup dry red wine
- Juice of 1 lemon
- 1 clove garlic, chopped

- Dried dill
- Chopped parsley
- Salt, pepper
- 2 lb monkfish

Add all the ingredients but the fish, plus ½ cup water to a large saucepan. Bring to a boil. Reduce the heat. Place the fish on top of the vegetables. Cover and cook 15 minutes longer. Arrange on a serving dish. Strain the sauce through a sieve and pour it over the fish. Serve immediately.

Equivalent sources of animal protein

4 ounces fish or shellfish (18 oysters or 24 mussels on average) = 4 ounces lean meat: veal, beef, game, lean pork tenderloin, rabbit, skinned poultry, offal (except duck and goose offal) = 2 slices of trimmed ham (4 ounces) = 2 eggs = 3 ounces hard cheese = 12 ounces low-fat plain yogurt or fromage frais = 6 ounces full-fat fromage frais

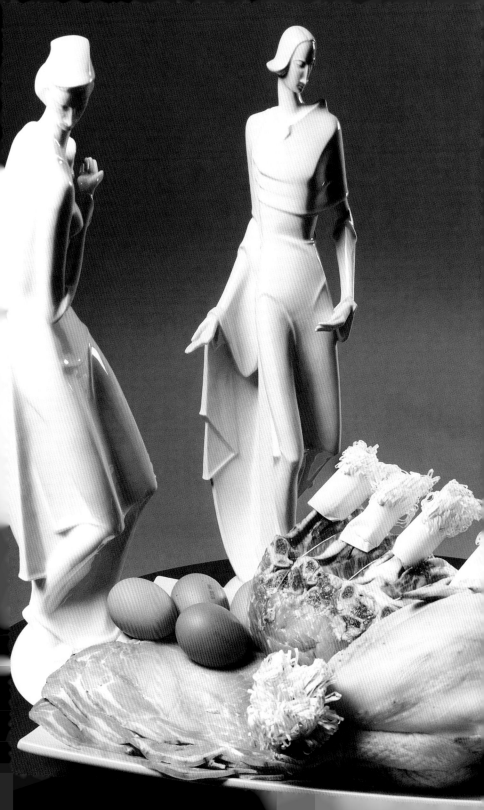

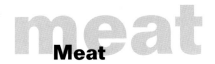

Meat

Veal with plums
Recipe for 6 (360 calories per serving)

- 4 shallots
- 1 tbsp light margarine
- 2 lb shoulder of veal, diced
- ½ cup dry white wine
- Salt, pepper
- 1 lb red plums

Peel and thinly slice the shallots. Melt the margarine in a saucepan. Gently sauté the shallots until golden. Add the veal and sauté until golden, stirring frequently and taking care that the shallots do not turn brown, as this would give them a bitter taste. Add the white wine. Season and mix together well. Cover and cook over very low heat for 50 minutes. Wash and dry the plums and add to the mixture. Cover and leave to simmer for 10 minutes longer before serving.

Turkey with peaches
Recipe for 6 (366 calories per serving)

- 8 peaches
- 4 shallots
- 2 tbsp light margarine
- ¾ cup dry white wine
- Salt, pepper
- 4 oz bacon, about 4 slices
- 1 small turkey, 6–7 lb

Place the peaches in a bowl and cover with boiling water. Leave for 5 minutes then drain, peel, split in two, and remove the pits. Peel and thinly slice the shallots. Preheat the oven to 450°F. Stuff the turkey with a mixture of the shallots, peaches, margarine, wine, salt, and pepper. Chop the bacon finely and place in a roasting dish with the turkey on top. Cook in the oven for 1 hour 50 minutes, basting and turning the turkey regularly.

Quail with huckleberries
Recipe for 4 (225 calories per serving)

- 8 oz huckleberries or blueberries
- 4 quail
- Salt
- 2 slices bacon, cut in half crosswise
- 4 sage leaves
- Kitchen string
- 2 tbsp light margarine
- ½ cup dry white wine

Remove the huckleberries from the stem and wash and drain. Stuff the quail with the huckleberries and season with salt. Arrange a strip of bacon over each quail. Slip a sage leaf inside and tie up with string. Melt the margarine in a saucepan and brown the quail on all sides. Pour the wine over, cover and leave to simmer for 15 minutes.

Ham and raspberry mousse
Recipe for 4 (415 calories per serving)
- 1 lb cooked ham
- 3 eggs
- Salt, pepper
- ½ cup low-fat crème fraîche
- 1 tbsp butter
- 6 oz raspberries

Finely chop or purée the ham. Break the eggs, season, and add to the ham with the crème fraîche. Preheat the oven to 350°F. Butter a gratin dish and place in it half the ham mixture, then the raspberries, then the rest of the ham. Smooth the surface well. Line a slightly larger ovenproof dish with wax or parchment paper and add water to a depth of about 1 inch. Place the dish containing the mousse in the water and bake for about 35 minutes. Serve hot or cold.

Uncovering the "hidden fat" in meat
In order to control your weight, the choice of meat is of prime importance, as their "hidden fat" content can vary between 5 and 25 percent according to the cut. It is therefore possible to make chili con carne using beef containing 5 percent fat, whereas the meat normally used for such dishes contains 15 or 20 percent fat. To retain a strong flavor it is important to add plenty of seasoning (tomatoes, Tabasco, onions, herbs, etc.). If the visible fat is removed from meat, certain fatty cuts become lean, as is the case with pork.

Roast veal with cherries
Recipe for 4 (473 calories per serving)
- 1 lb cherries
  (preferably not overripe)
- 2 onions
- 1 tbsp light margarine
- 1 lb veal roast
- Salt, pepper
- ¾ cup dry white wine

Wash the cherries and drain well. Thinly slice the onions. Melt the margarine in a saucepan. Brown the onions, then add the meat and brown on all sides, taking care not to let the onions burn. Season, add the wine, and turn the meat over. Cover and simmer over low heat for 50 minutes. Add the cherries and simmer for 10 minutes longer, uncovered.

Guinea fowl with cherries
Recipe for 4 (445 calories per serving)
- 16 cherries
- Salt, pepper
- 1 guinea fowl, about 2½ lb
- 3 tbsp light margarine
- 4 oz fresh mushrooms
- 8 shallots

Wash and dry the cherries. Season the guinea fowl. Melt the margarine in a large pan and brown the guinea fowl on all sides. Season. Add the cherries and cover. Cook for 15 minutes. During this time, clean the mushrooms. Chop the mushrooms and shallots and add to the pan. Cover and continue to cook for 50 minutes longer, turning the guinea fowl two or three times.

Veal cutlets with rosemary
Recipe for 2 (270 calories per person)
- Dried rosemary
- 12 oz veal cutlets
- Salt, pepper

Sprinkle rosemary over the cutlets to taste. Broil both sides close to the heat source. Season.

Rabbit with tomatoes
Recipe for 4 (308 calories per serving)
- 4 cloves of garlic, chopped
- 4 shallots, sliced
- 4 oz carrots, grated
- Chopped parsley
- Salt, pepper
- ½ cup white wine
- 1 young rabbit, cut into pieces, about 1 lb
- 1 tbsp chopped thyme
- 1 bay leaf
- 8 oz mushrooms, thinly sliced
- 12 oz tomatoes, peeled and chopped
- 5 tsp flour

Mix together the garlic, shallots, carrots, parsley, and pepper. Place in a saucepan, adding the white wine. Simmer, covered, for 10 minutes. Add the rabbit, thyme, bay leaf, and 1 cup water. Cook for 40 minutes. Halfway through this time add the mushrooms, tomatoes, and the flour made into a paste with a little cold water. Check the seasoning and serve.

Shish kebabs
Recipe for 2 (300 calories per serving)

- 10 oz lean lamb
- 1 onion
- Lemon slices
- Cherry tomatoes
- Thyme

Cut the meat into cubes and chop the onion into large pieces. Thread skewers alternately with lemon slices, onion pieces, tomatoes, and cubes of meat. Sprinkle with thyme. Broil for about 8 minutes, turning, until brown on all sides.

Which are the lean meats?
The lean meats are poultry—skinned chicken, guinea fowl, and turkey— and ham with visible fat removed. Offal is also very lean, apart from the brains and tongue. Eggs can also be used to replace meat, up to a maximum of 4–6 per week (they are included in many other products). As for seafood, all white fish and shellfish are low in fat.

Chicken with olives ⦂
Recipe for 4 (280 calories per serving)

- 1¼ lb chicken breast
- Salt, pepper
- Oil
- 12 oz carrots
- 12 oz onions
- 24 pitted green olives
- ¼ cup white wine
- ¼ cup vegetable stock
- Chopped parsley

Cut the chicken into pieces. Season. Brown in a little oil, turning once, until well browned on all sides. Drain on paper towels. Chop the carrots, slice the onion, and cook in boiling salted water. Drain. Add the chicken, vegetables, olives, wine, and vegetable stock to a saucepan. Bring to a boil and reduce for several minutes. Arrange on a serving dish and sprinkle with parsley.

Slow cooked dishes are beneficial—as long as they are correctly prepared

Watching what you eat does not mean depriving yourself of all culinary pleasures, particularly slow-cooked casseroles, one of the pleasures of winter. However, to avoid your weight suffering as a result, you should adapt traditional dishes with some of today's methods.

Remove all visible fat. Make low-fat sauces. The cooking method is also important. In order to reduce or completely eliminate the fat, stick to the oven (roasting, cooking in foil), the broiler, boiling (skimming off the fat if necessary), and the microwave.

Chicken breasts with cabbage leaves ⊙

Recipe for 4 (250 calories per serving)

- 5 chicken breast halves
- 4 oz low-fat fromage frais or plain yogurt
- 1 egg white
- Salt, pepper
- 8 oz mushrooms
- 1 cabbage
- 3 carrots, chopped
- 2 shallots, chopped
- 1 cup dry white wine
- 1 cup chicken stock
- 3 tbsp low-fat cream

Purée one chicken breast half, the fromage frais, and the egg white until they have reached the texture of a mousse. Season. Chop the mushrooms and mix ½ into the mousse. Separate the cabbage leaves and blanch in boiling water for about 3 minutes. Arrange one chicken breast half and a little mousse on 2 cabbage leaves and roll up. Repeat with the three other chicken breast halves. Steam for about 20 minutes. Meanwhile, prepare the sauce. Cook the carrots, shallots, and remaining mushrooms in the wine and stock. Reduce by half. Purée, then add the cream. Cook over low heat for 3 minutes. Pour into a serving dish and place the chicken breasts on top.

Quail flambé ⊙

Recipe for 4 (255 calories per serving)

- 8 quail
- 2 cups dry white wine
- Thyme
- Rosemary
- Salt, pepper
- 4 large oranges
- Juice of 1 lemon
- 1 liqueur glass of Grand Marnier

Remove the innards from the quail and clean thoroughly. Marinate for 24 hours in the wine and herbs. Drain, season, and cook in a hot oven for 10 minutes, basting frequently, until lightly browned. Squeeze the oranges and lemon (retain the orange halves). Pour the juice over the quail and cook for 5–10 minutes, basting frequently. Place each quail in the peel of half an orange. Bring the Grand Marnier to a boil, then pour over the quail and flambé. Serve the cooking liquids in a small pitcher or gravy boat.

Duck with mushrooms ⦿

Recipe for 4 (290 calories per serving)

- 1 duck
- 1 onion, chopped
- ½ cup red wine
- 1 bay leaf
- Juice of 1 lemon
- 8 oz mushrooms
- Basil
- Salt, pepper

Remove the duck fillets. Chop the carcass into pieces and brown in a saucepan with the onion. Pour off the excess fat and add the wine. Reduce until the liquid has evaporated completely. Add 2 cups water and the bay leaf, then cook for about 1 hour. In a different saucepan, pour the lemon juice over the whole mushrooms, add the basil and cook for about 5 minutes. Purée. Strain the liquid from the duck carcass through a sieve and reduce. Add the mushroom purée. Check the seasoning. Brown the duck fillets for 4 minutes each side in a nonstick frying pan. Pour the sauce over and serve.

Grilled lamb chops with mint ⦿

Recipe for 4 (350 calories per serving)

- 8 lamb cutlets
- Olive oil
- Mint

Brush the cutlets with a little oil. Leave to marinate for 20 minutes. Finely chop the mint, leaving a few leaves for garnish. Roll the cutlets in the mint on both sides. Broil. Serve garnished with mint leaves.

Calf's liver with wild strawberries
Recipe for 4 (216 calories per serving)
- 1 tbsp light margarine
- 4 slices calf's liver, about 4 oz each
- Salt, fresh ground black pepper
- Juice of 1 lemon
- 4 oz strawberries (wild if possible)

Melt the margarine in a frying pan and brown the liver on both sides, turning with a spatula, not with a fork as that might pierce the surface and cause the blood to escape. Total cooking time should not exceed 10 minutes. Season. Squeeze the lemon. Arrange the liver on a warm serving dish. Pour the lemon juice into the frying pan, add the strawberries, and stir gently with a spatula while they warm through. Pour around the liver and serve immediately.

Chicken with mushrooms and white wine
Recipe for 8 (255 calories per serving)
- 8 chicken breast halves
- 1 onion
- 1 tbsp olive oil
- ⅔ cup dry white wine
- Chopped parsley
- Basil
- 1 lb tomatoes, peeled and diced
- 4 oz mushrooms
- ¼ cup chicken stock

Skin the chicken breast halves. Chop the onion. Heat the oil in a frying pan and brown the onion and chicken pieces. Add the white wine, chopped parsley, basil, and tomatoes. Finely slice the mushrooms and add to the mixture with the chicken stock. Cover and cook over low heat for 10 minutes. Serve hot.

Braised lamb in wine sauce
Recipe for 6 (350 calories per serving)
- 2 lb leg of lamb
- Olive oil
- 2 cloves garlic, chopped
- 1 onion, chopped
- ½ cup dry red wine
- Rosemary
- ½ cup tomato purée

Finely dice the lamb and brown in the olive oil in a frying pan with the garlic and onion until golden brown. Add the wine, rosemary, and tomato purée then bring to a boil. Lower the heat and simmer for about 10 minutes. Add a little more tomato purée if necessary.

Steak flambé

Recipe for 4 (325 calories per serving)
- 1 tbsp olive oil
- 4 tsp low-fat butter
- 4 slices beef tenderloin
- ½ cup dry red wine
- Fresh ground black pepper
- 3 tbsp cognac

Heat the oil and butter in a frying pan and brown the meat. Pour in the wine and lower the heat, taking care not to overcook the meat. Season with pepper. Heat the cognac then pour over the cooked meat and flambé. Serve immediately, pouring the sauce over the steaks.

Roast guinea fowl with tarragon

Recipe for 4 (350 calories per serving)
- ½ cup nonfat milk
- 1 slice stale bread
- 1 cup shredded cheddar
- Chopped tarragon
- Salt, pepper
- 4 oz chicken liver
- 1 large guinea fowl, liver set aside
- ½ cup wine vinegar

Heat the milk and soak the bread in it. In a food processor, purée the cheese, tarragon, salt, pepper, chicken liver, and the liver of the guinea fowl and add the soaked bread. Stuff the guinea fowl with the mixture. Bake in a moderate oven for about 40 minutes. Baste from time to time with a little water mixed with the vinegar. Carve the guinea fowl into pieces before serving.

Carpaccio

Recipe for 4 (275 calories per serving)
- 1 lb whole beef tenderloin
- Juice of 2 lemons
- 2 tbsp olive oil
- Chopped parsley
- 1 tsp black pepper

Place the tenderloin in the freezer for 2 hours to make it easier to slice. Slice into very thin, almost transparent slices. Spread out over 4 plates. Mix the lemon juice, oil, parsley, and pepper together. Pour over the meat and serve.

Oven-baked veal chops ⊙

Recipe for 4 (260 calories per serving)

- 4 veal cutlets, 1 inch thick
- Thyme
- Salt, pepper
- ½ onion, finely sliced
- 1 clove garlic, chopped
- 2 stalks celery, finely sliced
- ½ cup dry white wine
- ½ cup chicken stock
- 2 tbsp cornstarch

Season the cutlets with the thyme, salt, and pepper. Arrange the meat, onion, garlic, and celery in an ovenproof dish. Add the wine and stock and cook, uncovered, in the oven for about 1 hour. Remove the cutlets and strain the sauce through a sieve, then thicken with the cornstarch. Pour over the cutlets.

Can game form part of a low-fat diet?

Game (pheasant, quail, venison, hare, pigeon, wild boar, etc.) has a low fat content of only 3 to 5 grams per 4 ounces. It is, however, particularly high in uric acid and is therefore not recommended for those who suffer from gout.

Flavor it with wine or beer; alcohol evaporates when cooked. Use fruit (blueberries, apples, grapes, pears), which goes well with game, and mushrooms. Create delicious marinades using red wine, onions, carrots, bay leaves, thyme, pepper, juniper berries, and cloves, which will permeate the meat and give a delightful flavor. It is also a good idea to use a stuffing based on low-fat yogurt or fromage frais. The meat will be even more tender and hardly any higher in fat content.

Entertaining

Throughout my life I have been fortunate enough to have the opportunity to taste dishes from all over the world. After trying practically everything, my aim now is to eat tasty food that is allowed on my diet so that I do not have to risk losing my newfound shape. My menus are designed with my doctor's advice in mind and I enjoy eating the delicious foods my chef prepares for me. I also appreciate his little discoveries, such as mixing my protein supplements with sauces, soups, or soufflés.

I have never eaten so much fish, poultry, or veal in my life and I feel wonderfully well on it. I wonder if I would still be capable of swallowing a rare sirloin steak. When I entertain, which I do frequently, my chef designs the menu in accordance with my doctor's advice. If the main course is not fish, he prepares me a separate portion. I drink my beloved Diet Pepsi with it and nobody notices anything strange.

K.L.

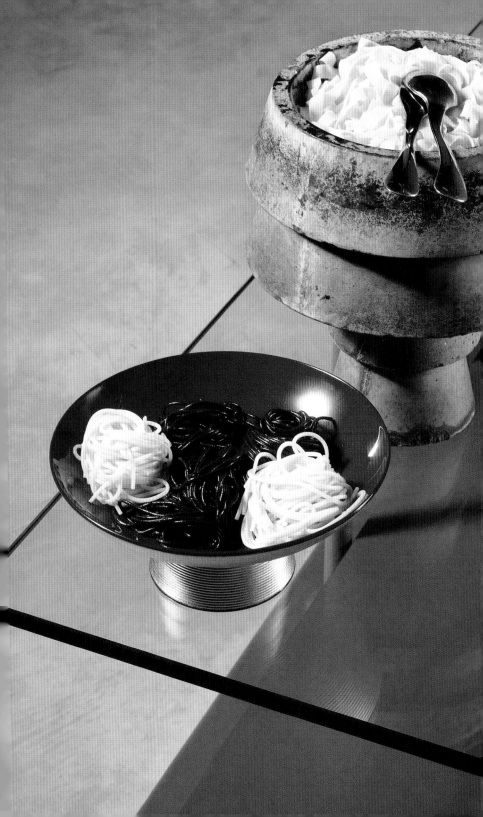

Pasta and pizza

Spaghetti with salmon ⊙
Recipe for 4 (380 calories per serving)
- 10 oz spaghetti
- 1 tbsp olive oil
- 1 zucchini, thinly sliced
- 16 sugar snap peas
- 12 cherry tomatoes
- Salt, pepper
- 4 thin slices smoked salmon, cut into wide strips
- 2 tbsp chopped parsley
- ½ tsp chopped basil
- ¼ cup grated parmesan

Cook the spaghetti until al dente. Keep warm. Add the olive oil to a saucepan of water. Add the vegetables and season. Cover and cook for 5 minutes. Drain and add to the hot pasta. Add the salmon strips, parsley, and basil. Let sit, covered, for one minute. Sprinkle with the cheese and serve.

Pasta with pesto sauce ⊙
Recipe for 4 (315 calories per serving)
- 10 oz dried pasta, any type
- 1 bunch basil
- 2 sprigs marjoram
- Olive oil
- ¼ cup parmesan
- Salt, pepper

Cook the pasta. During this time, place the basil and marjoram in the food processor. Add 1 tablespoon oil and purée. Continue in this way until you have a smooth mixture, using no more than 3 tablespoons oil. Add the parmesan and mix again, adding a spoonful of hot water if the sauce is too thick. Pour a little of the sauce into a large bowl. Add the drained pasta and mix well. Season. Just before serving add the rest of the sauce.

Grains: some equivalent measures
6 ounces potatoes = 6 ounces cooked couscous = 6 ounces cooked pasta = ¾ cup cooked white rice = 6 ounces cooked green beans = 1¼ cups cooked lentils = 2 ounces white bread = 174 calories

pizza

Pasta with seafood sauce ⦂

Recipe for 4 (105 calories per serving)

- 2 cloves garlic
- 3 shallots
- 2 tbsp olive oil
- Chopped parsley
- 2 tsp marinara sauce

- 10 oz shellfish
  (prawns, mussels, scallops, etc.)
- 1 tomato, chopped
- 10 oz cooked pasta, any type

Chop the garlic and shallots. Brown in the hot oil for a few minutes. Add the chopped parsley and marinara sauce. Add the shellfish and the chopped tomato and cook for 3 minutes. Pour the mixture over the cooked pasta and serve.

Pizza ⦂

Recipe for 6, as a starter, or 3, as a main course
(200 calories per serving)

- 8 egg whites
- 1 cup whole wheat flour
- 2 tsp grated parmesan
- 4 tsp fromage frais or plain yogurt
- Garlic powder

- Mushrooms
- Onions
- Green peppers
- Tomato sauce
- Mozzarella, thinly sliced

In a large bowl mix together the egg whites, flour, grated parmesan, fromage frais, and garlic powder. Pour into a 12-inch pizza mold. Bake for about 12 minutes. Leave to cool for 4 minutes. Thinly slice the mushrooms, onions, and green peppers. Spread the tomato sauce over the crust. Add some thin slices of mozzarella, then the vegetables, finishing with another layer of mozzarella. Bake in a hot oven for 10–15 minutes until the cheese is melted and golden.

The place of pasta in a diet

In principle, pasta is inadvisable in the weight loss phase of the Spoonlight diet, as are rice and couscous, because starchy foods are extremely dense in calories (in the form of carbohydrates). Thus, a 10 ounce portion of egg pasta contains 310 calories and a 10 ounce portion of brown rice about 330 calories, not counting the fat content of any sauce that accompanies it.

I do nevertheless recommend the consumption of boiled or steamed potatoes as part of the Spoonlight diet.

Once the consolidation phase has been reached, things are quite different. Pasta and carbohydrates can be reintroduced into the diet in moderate amounts. In the case of strenuous physical exercise, the consumption of carbohydrates is recommended on the day in question, in proportion to the calories expended, of course.

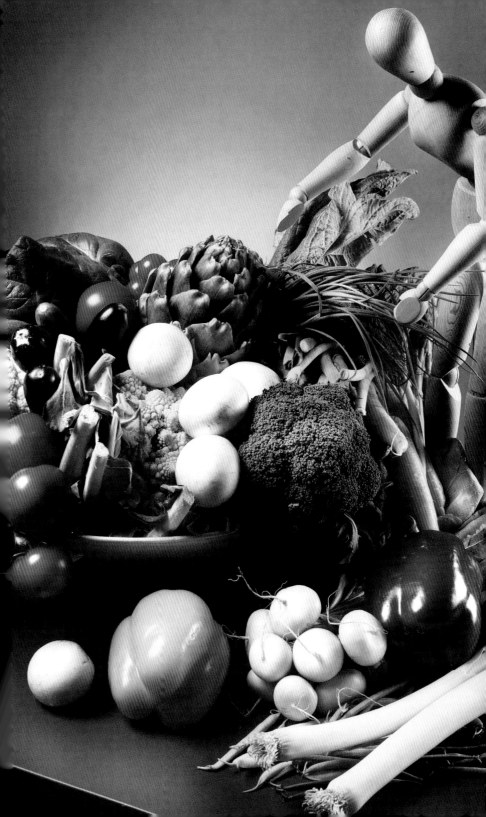

Vegetables

Stuffed endives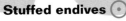
Recipe for 4 (80 calories per serving)
- 4 oz low-fat cream cheese
- 4 tsp crumbled Roquefort or blue cheese
- 2 tsp nonfat milk
- Salt, pepper
- 8 endive leaves per serving
- Paprika

In a bowl mix together the cream cheese, Roquefort, and milk, until you have a smooth paste. Season to taste. Fill each endive leaf with the mixture. Sprinkle with paprika. Serve cold.

Zucchini à la provençale
Recipe for 3 (65 calories per serving)
- 2 tbsp olive oil
- 2 cloves garlic, crushed
- 1 small onion, chopped
- 1 lb zucchini
- 1 tomato, diced
- 1 pinch thyme
- Salt, pepper

Heat the oil, then brown the crushed garlic and chopped onion. Slice the zucchini and add to the pan. Sauté gently for about 10 minutes until golden. Add the diced tomato and the thyme. Season. Cover and leave to cook for a further 35 minutes.

Stuffed artichokes
Recipe for 4 (206 calories per serving)
- 3 slices lean cooked ham
- 6 oz low-fat fromage frais or plain yogurt
- 1 egg
- ¼ cup gruyère or Swiss cheese
- Chopped parsley
- Salt, pepper
- 4 marinated artichoke hearts, drained

Finely chop the ham. Beat the fromage frais until smooth. Add the ham, the egg, two-thirds of the grated gruyère and the parsley. Season. Place the artichoke hearts in an ovenproof dish and spread the mixture over. Sprinkle with the remaining cheese. Bake for about 20 minutes.

Broccoli with tomato
Recipe for 4 (98 calories per serving)
- 2 lb broccoli
- 1 lb fresh tomatoes
- Salt, pepper
- 4 tsp grated parmesan
- 1 clove garlic, chopped
- Chopped parsley

Divide the broccoli into florets. Steam, then drain. Arrange in an ovenproof dish. Slice the tomatoes and arrange over the broccoli. Season. Sprinkle with the grated parmesan and garlic then bake in the oven. Immediately before serving, garnish with the chopped parsley.

Endives à la royale
Recipe for 4 (106 calories per serving)
- 2 lb endives
- 2 eggs
- ½ cup nonfat milk
- Salt, pepper

Wash the endives. Cook for 30 minutes in boiling salted water. Drain well. Beat the eggs with the milk. Season. Arrange the endives in an ovenproof dish and spread the mixture over. Bake in the oven until the eggs have set.

Creamed carrots
Recipe for 4 (187 calories per serving)
- 1 lb carrots
- 2 cups chicken stock
- ½ cup low-fat cream
- 1 egg yolk
- Chopped parsley
- Salt, pepper

Slice the carrots and cook in the chicken stock. Remove the carrots and arrange in an ovenproof dish. Reduce the stock and add the cream, egg yolk, and chopped parsley. Season. Pour the sauce over the carrots and reheat for a few minutes in the oven.

As many helpings of vegetables as you like
When following a protein diet, remember that you can eat unlimited quantities of the following vegetables (cooked without added fat): Swiss chard, broccoli, celery, mushrooms, cabbage, cucumbers, gherkins, zucchini, watercress, spinach, fennel, bean sprouts, mâche, peppers, radishes, lettuce.

The following vegetables, however, should be consumed in limited quantities (a maximum of half a pound per day): asparagus, eggplant, cardoons, cauliflower, endive, green beans, sorrel, tomatoes.

Spinach with prawns and rice
Recipe for 4 (220 calories per serving)

- 2 lb spinach
- 3 tbsp olive oil
- 20 medium prawns
- 4 cloves garlic, chopped
- ½ cup rice
- Salt

In a frying pan, cook the spinach for about 7 minutes in half the oil, then chop finely. Peel the prawns and prepare a stock with the shells and 3 cups water (or use purchased fish stock). Brown the chopped garlic and rice in the remaining oil. Add the spinach and the stock (twice as much stock as rice). Bring to a boil, then add the prawns and season. Once cooked, add more stock to thin if necessary.

Creamed cucumber
Recipe for 4 (85 calories per serving)

- 2 lb cucumbers
- 1 small onion, chopped
- ¼ cup low-fat cream
- Salt, pepper
- Chopped parsley

Peel the cucumbers and cut in half lengthwise. Remove the seeds. Cut into sticks. Steam for about 8 minutes. Drain well. During this time, heat the onion with the cream. Season. Add the cucumbers and simmer for 5 minutes. Sprinkle with parsley and serve immediately.

Three-vegetable terrine ⊙
Recipe for 8 (95 calories per serving)

- 2 lb carrots
- 2 lb cauliflower
- 1 lb green beans
- 3 egg whites
- Salt, pepper
- Fresh tomato coulis
  (see page 155)

Chop the carrots and break the cauliflower into florets. Steam the carrots, cauliflower, and beans separately. Purée each vegetable separately, adding an egg white to each one. Season. In a cake pan, spread a layer of carrot purée, then a layer of cauliflower purée, then a layer of bean purée. Place in a roasting pan of water and bake in a moderate oven for 45 minutes. Serve with fresh tomato coulis.

Leeks au gratin
Recipe for 4 (90 calories per serving)

- 8 leeks
- 4 eggs
- 1½ cups nonfat milk
- 1 tbsp gruyère or Swiss cheese
- Chopped parsley
- Salt, pepper

Wash the leeks thoroughly; steam then drain. Beat the eggs with the milk and gruyère. Add the chopped parsley. Place the leeks in an ovenproof dish. Pour the liquid over and place in the oven. Season. Bake on low heat for 4–5 minutes, then bake in a hot oven for a few more minutes. Serve immediately.

Vegetables in white sauce
Recipe for 4 (80 calories per serving)

- 1 lb cauliflower
- 10 oz broccoli
- 6 oz carrots
- Pinch thyme
- Salt, pepper
- 1 cup basic white sauce (see page 154)
- 2 tbsp butter
- 10 oz mushrooms, sliced
- 1 small onion, chopped
- ¼ cup grated cheese, such as gruyère or Swiss
- Paprika

Break the cauliflower and broccoli into florets. Steam separately until tender. Place on one side. Finely slice the carrots. Steam until tender. Add the thyme, salt, and pepper to the cooked cauliflower. Purée then mix in the white sauce until smooth. Melt the butter in a large saucepan and brown the sliced mushrooms and onion, stirring all the time. Add the carrots, broccoli, and sauce. Place in an ovenproof dish. Sprinkle with the cheese and paprika. Brown in the broiler.

Frozen and canned vegetables

Frozen vegetables have comparable nutritional value and vitamin content to fresh vegetables. Canned vegetables have comparable nutritional value but fewer vitamins. Take care, however, with precooked vegetables: always check the packet to see that the fat content does not exceed 5 grams per every 4 ounces.

Sautéed mushrooms ⊙

Recipe for 4 (50 calories per serving)

- Juice of 1 lemon
- 1 lb mushrooms
- 2 cloves garlic
- 1 tsp olive oil
- Chervil
- Ground coriander
- Salt, pepper

Squeeze the lemon. Clean and thinly slice the mushrooms. Sprinkle a little of the lemon juice over the mushrooms. Chop the garlic and brown in the olive oil. Add the mushrooms and cook for one minute, stirring. Add the rest of the lemon juice, the chervil, and the coriander. Season. Cover and cook for about 10 minutes. Serve hot or cold.

Vegetables in aspic ⊙

Recipe for 4 (60 calories per serving)

- 4 carrots
- 8 oz green beans
- 8 oz peas
- 2 stalks celery
- Salt, pepper
- 1½ packets unflavored gelatine

Cut the carrots in two, lengthwise. Trim the beans and remove any strings. Shell the peas. Dice the celery. Cook the vegetables in water, first the carrots, then the beans, peas, and celery. Retain 1¼ cups of the cooking water, season, and add the gelatine. Wait until it begins to set, then arrange the vegetables carefully in a mold. Pour the gelatine mixture over the vegetables. Chill for about 3 hours until set. Turn out and serve.

The advantages of vegetables

Although not a valuable source of energy, vegetables are packed with vitamins and minerals. Carrots, leeks, salsify, celery, fennel, endive, mushrooms, and turnips are particularly beneficial. Take care, however, with the quantity of fat used in the cooking and seasoning. Cabbage should not be forgotten, especially in stews or choucroute.

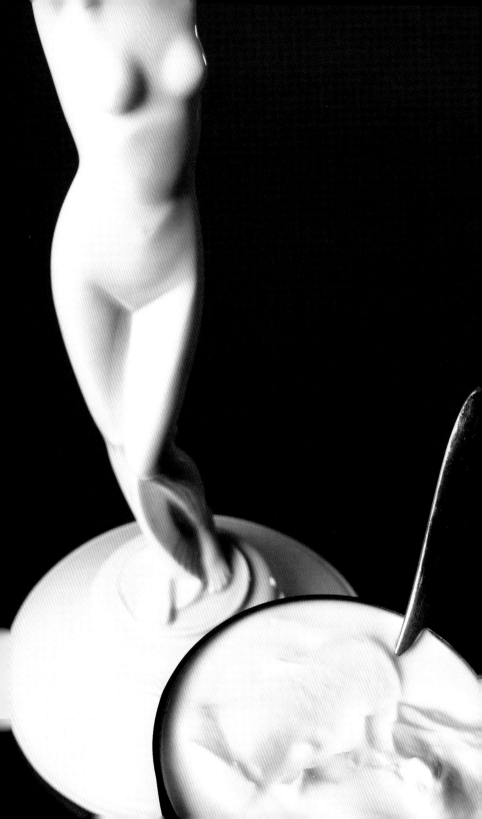

Sauces

Roquefort sauce ⊙
Recipe for 4 (100 calories per serving)
- 2 hard-boiled egg yolks
- 2 oz Roquefort or blue cheese
- 1 tbsp Dijon mustard
- 6 oz low-fat fromage frais or plain yogurt
- Olive oil
- Salt, pepper

Mix the egg yolks, Roquefort, and mustard to a paste. Beat the fromage frais until smooth. Mix all together. If the sauce is too thick add a little oil. Season to taste.

Yogurt sauce ⊙
Recipe for 4 (100 calories per serving)
- 1 plain yogurt
- 4 tbsp olive oil
- Juice of 1 lemon
- A hint of garlic
- Salt, pepper

Purée all the ingredients together. Check the seasoning. Serve cold.

Basic white sauce ⊙
Recipe for 8 (30 calories per serving)
- 2 tbsp cornstarch
- ¾ cup nonfat milk, heated
- Salt, pepper

Mix the cornstarch to a smooth paste in 2 tablespoons cold water. Add to the hot milk, stirring constantly until the mixture has thickened. Remove from heat. Season to taste.

Dishes with sauces: a matter of balance
In order to limit fat, it is important to look at a dish as a whole: a fatty piece of meat must be accompanied by a light sauce, whereas a lean piece of meat can be accompanied by a richer sauce. Meat served in a sauce can be less calorific than grilled meat if a lean cut of meat is chosen. Thus, a

4 ounce grilled steak can contain 14 grams fat, as compared to 9 grams for braised beef made from the blade-bone cut of beef shoulder, a moderately fatty cut of beef used for slow cooked dishes. Thus, stews and braised meats, in thick gravies and sauces, don't necessarily have to be high-fat; just choose a leaner cut of meat. Ask your butcher for other healthy suggestions.

Tarragon sauce
Recipe for 5 (55 calories per serving)

- 3 shallots
- ¼ cup vinegar
- ½ cup white wine
- 2 egg yolks

- 2 tbsp low-fat cream
- Coarsely chopped tarragon
- 2 pinches paprika
- Salt, pepper

Finely chop the shallots and brown in a saucepan. Add the vinegar and white wine. Reduce to half the volume. Remove from the heat and mix in the egg yolks, cream, tarragon, paprika, salt, and pepper. Mix until smooth.

Red wine sauce
Recipe for 4 (60 calories per serving)

- 1 onion
- 2 carrots
- 2 cups dry red wine

- 1½ tbsp butter
- Salt, pepper

Chop the onion and carrots. Cook in the red wine and allow the liquid to reduce by half, removing any froth that comes to the surface. Purée the vegetables in a food processor and return to the pan. Add the butter a little at a time until melted and well incorporated. Season. Serve with red meat.

Fresh tomato coulis ⊙
Recipe for 4 (60 calories per person)

- 1 lb fresh tomatoes
- 1 onion, chopped
- 2 cloves garlic, chopped
- Oregano
- Thyme

- Basil
- Tabasco
- 1½ tbsp butter
- Salt, pepper

Pour boiling water over the tomatoes and leave for 2 minutes. Plunge in cold water then remove the skins. Halve, seed, then dice. Brown the onion and garlic in a nonstick pan with a little water. Add the tomatoes, oregano, thyme, basil, and Tabasco and cook over moderate heat for about 10 minutes. Add the butter a little at a time. Season. Strain before use.

Cucumber sauce ⊙
Recipe for 8–10 (45 calories per serving)
- 1 large cucumber
- ¼ cup nonfat milk
- 2 tsp Dijon mustard
- 4 oz ricotta
- Chopped dill
- Salt, pepper

Peel the cucumber, slice lengthwise and remove the seeds, then chop. Purée the cucumber, milk, and mustard. Add the ricotta and mix until smooth. Add the dill and season. Chill to let the sauce thicken.

Mustard and fromage frais sauce ⊙
Recipe for 8 (30 calories per serving)
- 8 oz fromage frais or plain yogurt
- 3 tbsp whole-grain mustard
- Pinch paprika
- Salt, pepper
- Chopped parsley

Beat the fromage frais until creamy. Add the other ingredients and mix until smooth. Serve with fish or seafood.

How to cook sauces
Always use low-fat products (15 percent crème fraîche, low-fat butter, or light margarine). Use unlimited quantities of veal, chicken, or meat stock, adding no more than 5 grams fat per person. Unsweetened evaporated milk can be used to replace crème fraîche, as it contains three times less fat and is ideal for making low-fat sauces.

Pink sauce ⊙
Recipe for 8 (20 calories per serving)
- 8 oz fromage frais or plain yogurt
- Paprika
- 1 tsp wine vinegar
- Salt, pepper

Beat fromage frais until creamy, then stir in the other ingredients. Serve with fish or seafood.

Low-fat mayonnaise
Recipe for 8 (45 calories per serving)
- 2 eggs, separated
- 1 tbsp Dijon mustard
- 1 plain yogurt
- tbsp olive oil
- Salt, pepper

Hard-boil one of the eggs. Remove the yolk and mix it with the raw egg yolk. Mix with the mustard and yogurt and add the oil, drop by drop, stirring constantly. Season to taste. Serve with cold meat or fish.

Light béarnaise sauce ⊙
Recipe for 8 (25 calories per serving)
- Chives
- ½ cup wine vinegar
- Tarragon, parsley, salt, and pepper
- 2 egg yolks, beaten
- Pinch cayenne
- ¾ cup nonfat milk, boiling

Chop the chives. Cook in a nonstick pan with the vinegar, tarragon, parsley, salt, and pepper and reduce until the liquid has almost completely evaporated. Add the beaten egg yolks and the cayenne. Pour in the boiling milk, stirring constantly. Cook over very low heat, stirring constantly until the sauce has thickened. Serve hot with grilled meat.

Light sauces
Low-fat béchamel sauce can be made by stirring cornstarch directly into a little warm nonfat milk. Season with nutmeg, salt, and pepper. Mustard is also a staple and is excellent with any red meat, as are dried parsley, garlic, dill, and basil, to accompany meat, fish, or vegetable dishes. Delicious sauces can also be made with tomatoes, peppers, eggplant, etc.

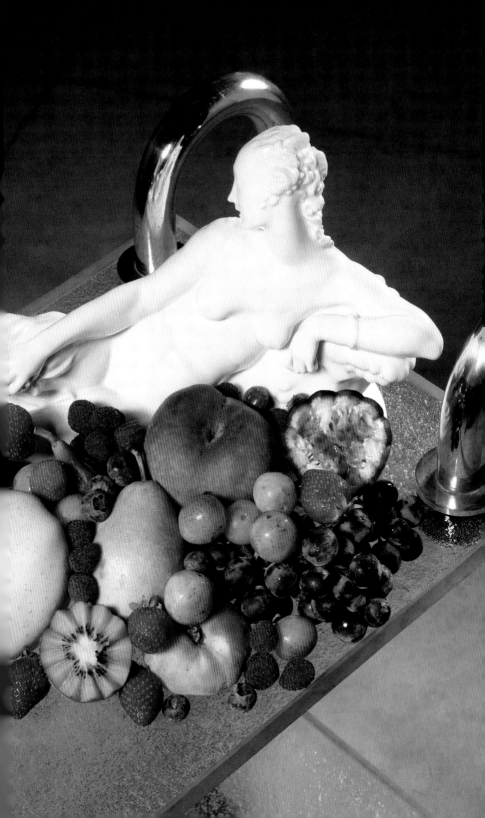

desserts

Desserts

Pomegranate sorbet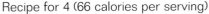
Recipe for 4 (116 calories per serving)

- 1⅓ lb pomegranates, halved
- Juice of 1 lemon
- ½ cup powdered artificial sweetener
- 2 egg whites

Squeeze the pomegranates by pressing the halves on a citrus juicer. Pour the pomegranate and lemon juice into a saucepan with all but 2 teaspoons of the sweetener. Bring to a boil and cook for 2 minutes. Cool. Beat the egg whites until stiff, gradually adding the rest of the sweetener. Fold the beaten egg whites carefully into the juice mixture. Pour into a suitable dish and freeze.

Strawberry and rhubarb compote
Recipe for 4 (66 calories per serving)

- 2 lb rhubarb
- 8 oz strawberries
- ¼ cup powdered artificial sweetener

Wash the rhubarb stalks and cook with 2 tablespoons water over very low heat, stirring frequently. Wash and hull the strawberries. When the rhubarb is cooked, chop and add the strawberries, leaving on the heat for only a few seconds so that the strawberries remain firm. Add the artificial sweetener. Cool, then chill. Serve very cold.

Strawberry mousse
Recipe for 6 (200 calories per serving)

- 1 lb strawberries
- ¾ cup granular sugar substitute
- Juice of 1 lemon
- 4 egg whites

Put 3 large strawberries aside for garnish. Hull the others and leave to soak in 2 ounces of the sugar and the lemon juice, then purée. Beat the egg whites until stiff, gradually adding the rest of the sweetener. Gently fold into the strawberry purée. Chill for 15 minutes. Decorate with slices of fresh strawberry. Serve immediately.

Fruit crêpes
Recipe for 4 (180 calories per serving)

Crêpes:
- ½ cup nonfat milk
- ½ cup flour
- 2 eggs, lightly beaten
- Salt
- Butter

Filling:
- 8 oz strawberries, hulled
- 1 banana
- Lemon juice
- 2 oz artificial sweetener

Crêpes: Gradually mix the milk into the flour, stirring constantly. Add the beaten eggs and mix well together. Add a pinch of salt. Cook the very thin crêpes in a little butter in a nonstick frying pan.

Filling: Cut the strawberries and banana into small pieces. Soak in the lemon juice and sweetener then use to fill the crêpes. Serve.

Raspberry coulis
Recipe for 4 (20 calories per serving)
- 10 oz raspberries
- Juice of 1 lemon
- Artificial sweetener

Purée the raspberries and lemon juice together. Add artificial sweetener to taste. Strain through a sieve. Serve very cold.

Fruit sweetmeats
Recipe for 3 dozen sweetmeats (25 calories per sweetmeat)
- 4 oz pitted prunes
- 4 oz raisins
- 4 oz pitted dates
- ¼ cup shredded coconut

Mix the prunes, raisins, dates, and coconut together in a bowl. Boil in a little water for about 10 minutes. Crush all together with a pestle and mortar or briefly pulse in a food processor. Shape into small balls, 1 inch in diameter. Chill for about 2 hours. Serve.

Fruit in all its forms

Fruit is available all year round, even in winter, especially citrus fruits (oranges, grapefruit, clementines), which are rich in vitamin C (a large orange provides the recommended daily amount), apples, and pears. There are also tropical fruits (kiwifruit, pineapples, litchis, mangoes, papayas). If you like stewed fruit, eat it plain or with a teaspoon of powdered sugar or artificial sweetener. Look for canned fruit in juice, not syrup.

Crème pâtissière ☺

Recipe for 6 (95 calories per serving)

- ⅓ cup cornstarch
- 2 cups nonfat milk
- ⅓ cup vanilla sugar
- 2 tbsp Cointreau

Mix the cornstarch to a paste in a little cold milk. Bring the rest of the milk and sugar to a boil, stirring constantly. Add the cornstarch and bring to a boil, stirring constantly. Flavor with the liqueur. Serve the custard as it is after leaving in the fridge for 1 hour or use to line the base of a fruit tart.

Almond ring ☺

Recipe for 6 (195 calories per serving)

- ¾ cup sifted flour
- ½ cup sugar
- 1 cup ground almonds
- 10 egg whites
- Pinch salt
- 1 tsp vanilla extract
- A few drops of orange extract

Preheat the oven to 250°F. Sift the flour in two parts, half with half the sugar and the other half with the ground almonds. Set aside. Beat the egg whites with the pinch of salt until stiff. Add the vanilla and orange extract. Add the rest of the sugar a little at a time, alternating with small amounts of the two flour mixtures. When everything has been mixed together, pour into an ungreased ring-shaped mold. Bake for 30 minutes, until golden. Turn out and cool.

Desserts: a few ground rules

Even when on a diet, desserts should be a treat. Don't cut out this essential part of life's pleasures, but do indulge in moderation. One helping of sweet crêpes, for example, contains as much fat as three tablespoons of oil! On a daily basis, stick to fruit and dairy products. If you think that you may be tempted by a rich dessert, take care to keep down the fat content of the rest of your meal.

Mocha petits fours
Recipe for 24 petits fours (37 calories each)

- ⅓ cup light margarine
- 2 tbsp brown sugar
- ¼ cup sugar
- ¾ cup sifted flour
- 2 egg yolks (duck eggs if possible)
- ¼ cup unsweetened cocoa powder
- 2 tsp instant coffee granules
- 1 tsp dried yeast
- Pinch salt

Preheat the oven to 200°F. Beat the margarine, brown sugar, and sugar on full speed in a food processor until creamy. Add the sifted flour, egg yolks, cocoa, instant coffee, yeast, and salt. Mix well. Arrange small mounds of the mixture on a nonstick baking sheet. Bake for about 15 minutes.

Chocolate minarets
Recipe for 4 (186 calories per serving)

Base:
- 3 tbsp light margarine
- ½ cup sifted flour
- Pinch dried yeast
- 2 eggs

Filling:
- 2 tbsp nonfat milk
- ¼ cup unsweetened cocoa powder
- 2 oz low-fat fromage frais or plain yogurt
- 2 tbsp sugar

Base: Preheat the oven to 250°F. Bring ¼ cup water and the margarine to a boil in a saucepan. Add the flour and yeast. Stir the mixture until it comes away from the sides of the pan then leave on the heat for another 30 seconds. Remove from the heat, add the eggs one by one, and mix until well blended. On a greased baking sheet make 4 small mounds, using 2 spoonfuls of the mixture for each and hollowing out the inside of each one.

Bake for 20 minutes. Cool.

Filling: Heat the milk and cocoa powder in a saucepan, stirring constantly. Remove from the heat and add the fromage frais and sugar, stirring constantly. Cool, then put in the fridge. Cut off the top of each mound, fill with the chocolate cream, and replace the top.

Raspberry sorbet ⊙

Recipe for 4 (96 calories per serving)

- 1 lb raspberries
- Juice of 1 lemon
- ½ cup artificial sweetener
- 1 tsp raspberry liqueur

Set aside 12 large raspberries. Press the rest of the raspberries through a sieve to obtain juice. Mix together the raspberry juice, lemon juice, sweetener, and liqueur. Pour into a sorbet maker or suitable dish. Freeze. (If using a sorbet maker, follow manufacturer's instructions.) Immediately before serving, garnish each serving with 3 raspberries.

Meringue cups ⊙

Recipe for 4 (45 calories per serving)

- Pinch salt
- 2 egg whites
- 2 tbsp powdered sugar
- 8 oz unsweetened applesauce
- Zest of 1 lemon

Add the salt to the egg whites. Beat until the mixture stands up in peaks. Using a spatula, fold in the sugar, applesauce, and lemon zest. Divide between 4 glasses. Chill for 5 hours.

Fruit delight ⦙

Recipe for 4 (138 calories per serving)

- 2 egg whites
- 2 tbsp powdered sugar
- 2 tsp salt
- 4 oz hulled strawberries
- 1 lb canned peaches

Beat the egg whites, half the sugar, and the salt with an electric hand mixer until firm. Using a spoon, drop 16 small meringues onto a baking sheet. Pour the rest of the sugar into a saucepan full of water. Bring to a boil then lower the heat. Plunge the meringues into the water 4 at a time. Leave in the water for 4 minutes, then drain. Purée the strawberries and peaches in their juice for 5 seconds. Divide the purée between 4 glasses and decorate each one with 4 meringues. Store chilled.

Beware of dried fruit

Dried fruit (dates, figs, apricots, prunes, etc.) and nuts (walnuts, hazelnuts, almonds) are a source of minerals but must be eaten in moderation as they both have a high sugar content, and nuts are also high in fat.

Jellied fruit terrine

Recipe for 4 (110 calories per serving)

- 1 slice watermelon
- 1 papaya
- Juice of 1 lemon
- 8 oz blackberries

- 8 oz raspberries
- 2 oz artificial sweetener
- 1 packet unflavored gelatine

Seed the watermelon and dice the flesh. Cut the papaya in two, remove the pit, and dice the flesh. Squeeze the lemon. Set aside 10 large blackberries. Purée the others, then strain to remove the seeds. Do the same with the raspberries (setting aside 10). In a bowl mix together the juices of the lemon, blackberries, and raspberries; add the sweetener. Bring to a boil. Add the gelatine to the juice, stirring constantly until dissolved, and bring back to a boil. Remove from the heat. Rinse a fruit bowl in cold water and pour in half of the juice/gelatine mixture. Leave until semicooled. Arrange the watermelon cubes, papaya cubes, whole blackberries, and raspberries over the jelly, which will begin to set. Slowly pour over the remaining juice/gelatine mixture. When completely cooled, chill for 4–10 hours.

Good ways to use artificial sweeteners and different types of sugar

The systematic use of sweeteners containing aspartame is recommended when preparing desserts. For best results, sweeten generously with aspartame after cooking as its sweetening power is released by heat. You can also use fructose, which has the advantage of being a natural product, but which provides more calories for the same amount of sweetening power.

When not on a strict weight loss diet it is often a good idea to use powdered sugar for decoration. It is high in calories but, because it is so light and fine, a very small amount goes a long way.

Fruit salad with red berries
Recipe for 4 (70 calories per serving)

- 8 oz strawberries, hulled
- 8 oz raspberries
- 8 oz blackberries

- 8 oz red currants
  or more raspberries
- ½ cup orange juice

Cut the strawberries into thick slices. Put the berries and the currants into a bowl and add the orange juice. Chill for 2 hours before serving.

Lemon mousse
Recipe for 6 (230 calories per serving)

- 6 eggs
- 10 oz sugar

- Juice of 3 lemons
- Zest of 1 lemon

Put the eggs, sugar, lemon juice, lemon zest, and 1 cup water in a saucepan. Beat together. When the mixture is frothy, place the saucepan over another saucepan containing hot water and continue to beat until the mixture just comes to a boil. Pour the mousse into a serving dish and continue to beat for another 5 minutes. Cool.

Keep an eye on your chocolate consumption
If you are a "chocoholic" don't cut it out of your diet completely. It is better to get into the habit of eating in moderation. Don't eat more than 1 ounce per day, or a medium-sized bar of chocolate. Try to eat it with bread or toast to retain some balance. If you eat chocolate on its own you risk consuming much more of it. Avoid chocolate with nuts (almonds, walnuts, hazelnuts) as well as truffles and filled chocolates. It is also important to remember that the more cocoa butter the chocolate contains, the higher the fat content. So-called "diet chocolate" is therefore often more fattening than normal chocolate. And don't overlook artificially sweetened chocolates.

Dairy products: the happy medium

For a diet containing sufficient calcium, some dairy is recommended at each meal. Low-fat products are ideal. In the weight loss phase of the diet, limit yourself to low-fat fromage frais or plain yogurt, and in the next phase just one small portion of cheese per day. Desserts containing fruit and dairy products are recommended, such as a bowl of fromage frais with pears or kiwifruit.

Sweet things

Despite the fact that I grew up during the war, our cook used to make big, creamy, sweet, German cakes. Indeed, milk, butter, and cream exist in unlimited quantities in northern Germany. But even then I wasn't too fond of that type of cake, which was certainly nice but rather over the top. I always preferred less sweet things such as pancakes, waffles, shortbread, etc. Nowadays I never fancy that type of thing. On my doctor's orders, I regularly eat fresh or stewed fruit, despite the fact that I don't really like it very much.

K.L.

1- Jo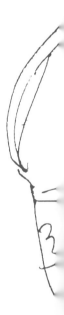

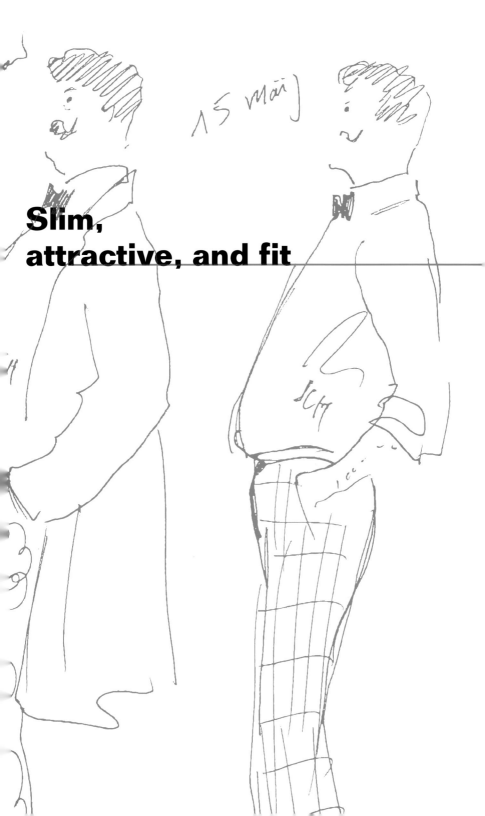

Slim,
attractive, and fit

Becoming slim and remaining slim: undoubtedly a most enticing proposition.…But just getting their figure back is not always enough to satisfy my patients. Many of them also want to look healthier and to lead a more active life on all fronts: sports, work, sex.…In short, they want to give themselves the best chance of starting a new life. Unfortunately, biological age and the effects of aging are still there and remind people that, however much they may have slimmed down, they are no longer twenty years old. This is all the more difficult to come to terms with in a society that persists in denying the possibility of either weight gain or aging.

Moreover (and whatever a patient's state of mind or however strong the desire for a youthful appearance is), weight loss can lead to a certain slackening of the features, and of the skin in general, particularly on the stomach, arms, buttocks, and hips.

Whether you wish to lose weight or merely look younger, there are solutions. In fact, there are several alternatives, some of which involve the latest medical and surgical advances. We shall go through the various treatments and techniques and their pros and cons.

Firstly, there are cosmetic treatments that aim to maintain, improve, and nourish the skin and to prevent the formation of wrinkles. These aim to give a healthier appearance and to cover up skin imperfections (through injections of vitamins or trace elements, or skin peeling using products ranging from phenol to fruit acids, according to the desired effect) and to reduce the appearance of wrinkles (through Botox injections and electrical impulse therapy).

Next, there is cosmetic surgery, which can involve the face (full or partial face-lift, liposuction to remove double chins, reshaping of facial contours, hair implants) and the body (reduction of residual excess fat through liposuction or liposculpture, reduction of loose skin on the stomach, inner thighs, arms, etc.). Thanks to cosmetic surgery, it is also possible to reduce the size of the breasts, which may still be too large even after a diet, and to correct drooping breasts (possibly with the use of an implant to restore both shape and size).

Finally, there are general treatments such as vitamins, minerals, anti-oxidants, and hormone replacement therapy.

This chapter would be incomplete without mentioning the adjustments that every individual should make to their daily life in order to regain—and to maintain—the peak of fitness after a diet. For this reason I feel that it is essential to mention healthy living, stress management, giving up smoking, and exercise (simple but very effective for those who are prepared to spend fifteen minutes a day to feel good about their bodies).

Because, if you wish to regain a self-image that allows you both to feel well and to match your external appearance with the man or woman you now feel yourself to be, science is certainly a great help but is not enough on its own: the search for a sense of balance, the desire to maintain a healthy body and a healthy mind—these are the keys to fitness and well-being.

Cosmetic treatments

For some years I have been aware of the effects of aging and dieting on the skin. There are plenty of remedies on the market but none of them were perfect for me, so I decided to create a range of products made from essential oils, vegetable extracts, and marine elements. These products are manufactured near the coast in small quantities in order to ensure maximum freshness and efficacy.

The active ingredients

The main active ingredients of this range of treatments are as follows:

Arbutin—an extract of bearberry (*Arbutus uva ursi*). This substance is a natural precursor of hydroquinone, which has long been known for its action against problems of pigmentation and age spots. We feel that the use of this substance in our cosmetic products is a guarantee of quality and uniform results.

Azulene—a natural balm extracted from the tropical plant gurjun, which is rich in oil resins. It is used in cosmetic treatments because of its softening effect on the skin.

Shea butter—extracted from the African tree *Butyrospermum parkii*. Shea butter is well known and much used for its healing powers and especially for its ability to penetrate the epidermis. It contains many fatty acids, the efficacy of which explains its success.

Marine collagen—one of the main constituents of collagen, the advantages of which are well known. When the collagen content of the skin is reduced, the thickness, firmness, and elasticity are also reduced and wrinkles appear.

Sea water—contains the same essential elements as blood plasma. The collagen from marine products is also very close to human collagen, which is why it is particularly beneficial in the prevention of wrinkles.

Consound—(*Symphytum officinale*) known since early times for its healing powers on bone fractures, cuts, and sores. This plant contains large amounts of allantoin, known for its healing powers, and anti-inflammatory phenols. Consound oil is used successfully for the treatment of acne and skin dehydration; its use in cosmetology is therefore particularly desirable.

Watercress and arugula—watercress (*Nasturtium officinale*) and arugula (*Eruca sativa*) contain high levels of vitamins A, B1, and B2 and mineral salts (iodine, iron, phosphate) but they owe their remarkable antioxidant effect to their exceptionally high vitamin C and E content. They are essential elements in anti-aging treatments.

Rose hips—the high vitamin C content of rose hips (the fruit of the dog rose) and the presence of anti–free radical elements makes this an essential component in anti-aging products.

Incense—incense has the power to regulate the secretion of oil by the sebaceous glands and is widely used in products for oily skin.

Fucus vesiculosus* and *Laminaria digitata—As with all types of seaweed, these are rich in elements derived from the ocean in which they live. They contain a concentrated cocktail of trace elements— copper, chromium, zinc, selenium, iron, manganese, and iodine—that are easily absorbed by the skin. They also contain, in their natural state, numerous vitamins including folic acid, vitamin C, and the B group vitamins (B1, B2, B6, and B12).

Guarana—this plant (*Paullinia cupana*) from the Amazonian forest contains large amounts of tannins, saponins, and especially caffeine and its relatives, theophylline and theobromine. Caffeine and its derivatives act on the cells by attacking reserves of fat and stimulating the circulation and flow of blood through the cells. This plant is very useful in anticellulite treatments.

Shark liver oil—used in cosmetic treatments because it is exceptionally rich in omega-3 fatty acids and vitamins A and E. It is an excellent ingredient in anti-aging products.

Wheat germ oil—the oil extracted from wheat germ (*Triticum sativum*) contains fat-soluble lipids and vitamins. The lipids consist mainly of essential fatty acids that help the body fight excess cholesterol and the hardening of the arteries. This oil is used in cosmetic preparations because of its high vitamin E content and its ease of absorption by the skin. Vitamin E is a powerful agent in the fight against free radicals and is therefore a precious ingredient in anti-aging preparations.

Oil of musk rose (*Rosa moschata*) and oil of kukui (*Aleutrites moluccana*)—kukui is an exotic plant from the Molluque islands. These oils contain large amounts of essential fatty acids. They have a particular ability to penetrate the skin and are widely used in cosmetic preparations for dry skin.

Essential oils of lavender, mint, rosemary, thyme, and oregano—the essential oils of aromatic plants are used in small doses in cosmetic preparations for their antiseptic, antibacterial, anti-fungal, soothing, and revitalizing properties.

Essential oils of orange, lemon balm, and eucalyptus—these essential oils are used in cosmetic preparations because of their decongestant and relaxing virtues.

Ispaghul—ispaghul seed (*Plantago ovata*) is rich in mucilage which, when combined with water, forms a natural gel. It is used in cosmetic preparations to manufacture natural gels to which different plant extracts can be added.

Ivy—ivy (*Hedera helix*) has long been known for its capacity to protect the surface of the skin. It is used successfully in the fight against cellulite and fatty deposits beneath the skin. It also has astringent and toning properties.

Lithothamnium calcareum—a type of seaweed containing concentrated elements of sea water. It is rich in calcium, magnesium, iron, and minerals. It protects the skin and guards against yeast and fungal infections of the candida type, which are often at the root of mycosis or thrush.

Horse chestnut—The horse chestnut tree (*Aesculus hippocastanum*) is known all over the world for its ability to treat hemorrhoids due to its ability to strengthen the lining of the veins. We use this plant in cosmetic preparations because of its ability to tone the small blood vessels beneath the skin.

St. John's wort—St. John's wort (*Hypericum perforatum*) is well known as an antidepressant. In cosmetic preparations it is used in the form of a red oil with antiseptic and toning properties.

Micronized olive pits—this fine powder made from crushed olive pits is used in exfoliating creams and lotions.

Propolis—a gluelike substance gathered by bees from tree bark. In the hive, propolis serves as cement to construct the framework of the cells of the honeycomb. Propolis protects against microbes, bacteria, and fungal infections, both in the hive and in cosmetic products.

Tepescohuite—this extract of *Mimosa tenuiflora* possesses strong skin healing and conditioning powers. In cosmetic preparations it is used particularly in conditioning and protective lotions.

Red grape vine—the leaves of red grape vines (*Vitis vinifera*) contain substances that are very beneficial to the skin:
• Anthocyanins, rich in vitamin B3, which act on the small blood vessels to make them more permeable.
• Tannins, which stimulate the tonicity of the small blood vessels.
• Proanthocyanidols, which protect the collagen of the small blood vessels against free radicals.

In cosmetic preparations the red grape vine is of great importance in the prevention and treatment of problems linked to ailments of the micro–blood vessels.

The products in the Basiques du Manoir line

We have created a line of products to moisturize and treat all types of skin, as well as specific products for dark skin. The use of these cosmetics reduces the signs of aging and the slackening of skin. The line is comprehensive and includes:

Anti-aging face and body lotions

• **Sun Papaya Q10 Face Cream**—this cream is full of papaya extract, ceramides, and coenzyme Q10 and is specifically adapted to prevent the sagging of facial tissue and wrinkle formation. Begin this treatment before wrinkles first appear. If wrinkles are already present this treatment will ameliorate their appearance.

• **Sun Papaya Q10 Body Cream**—this cream contains a good amount of papaya extract, ceramides, and coenzyme Q10. Its formula is specifically suited to improve the tonicity and elasticity of the skin. This treatment is of particular use during and after a slimming diet for people whose skin lacks tonicity and for women during and after pregnancy.

Moisturizing face lotions

• **Gommage Douceur (Gentle Scrub)**—this nonabrasive exfoliating cream has a deep cleansing effect, removing dead cells and brightening the complexion. It works simply through contact with the skin and is particularly suitable for very sensitive skin (ingredients: lithothame, starch).

• **Sérum Tenseur (Firming Cream)**—a concentrate of active ingredients that gives the skin a youthful glow (ingredients: marine collagen, tepescohuite, moisturizing vegetable extract, protein).

• **Crème Réparatrice (Repairing Cream)**—very fragile and sensitive skin occasionally requires a very rich lotion. This cream contains extract of *Mimosa tenuiflora* and propolis, whose conditioning properties are self-evident (ingredients: excipient, wheat germ oil, shea butter, oil of musk rose, oil of kukui, propolis, *Mimosa tenuiflora*, zinc oxide, allantoin).

• **Masque Douceur (Gentle Mask)**—skin requires deep treatment and care once a week. This mask provides essential nutrients (ingredients: wheat germ oil, shea butter, oil of musk rose, oil of kukui, shark liver oil, marine collagen, moisturizing vegetable extract, allantoin, zinc oxide).

• **Lait Démaquillant (Cleansing Lotion)**—its main purpose is to eliminate all skin impurities such as makeup, excess oil, grime, and dead cells. It should be used twice a day (morning and night). This cleansing lotion is very gentle and both protects and cleanses thoroughly (ingredients: excipient, wheat germ oil, concentrate of vegetable protein, seaweed extract, ivy extract).

• **Lotion Douceur (Gentle Lotion)**—use after the Lait Démaquillant to remove it completely (ingredients: extracts of seaweed, ivy, and mimosa, vegetable protein concentrate).

- **Crème de Nuit (Gentle Night Cream)**—richer and therefore more nourishing than the day creams, it complements them and maximizes their potential (ingredients: wheat germ oil, shea butter, oil of musk rose, oil of kukui, shark liver oil, marine collagen, moisturizing vegetable extract, allantoin).

- **Crème Plein Air (Outdoor Cream)**—certain types of skin require a particularly high level of daily protection and nourishment; the special Crème Plein Air provides that. This oil-rich cream acts as sunblock. It should be used from time to time by those who work outdoors, and regularly by those with particularly delicate skin (ingredients: wheat germ oil, shea butter, oil of musk rose, oil of kukui, *Mimosa tenuiflora*, moisturizing marine extract, allantoin, sunscreen, carotene).

- **Sérum Clarifiant pour les Peaux Tachées (Clarifying Serum)**—a concentrate of nourishing active ingredients that maximizes the effects of the creams and mask (ingredients: excipient, seaweed extract, arbutin).

- **Crème Contour des Yeux (Eyes Contour Cream)**—the skin around the eyes is very fine and delicate, requiring regular, specific care. This special eye cream protects the epidermis against premature aging (ingredients: wheat germ oil, shea butter, oil of musk rose, oil of kukui, *Mimosa tenuiflora*, moisturizing marine extract, moisturizing vegetable extract, ivy extract, hyaluronic acid).

Specific treatment lotions

- **Oily skin line**—this includes a facial scrub with absorbent properties (ingredients: wheat germ oil, extracts of propolis, rosemary, seaweed, lavender, incense, natural exfoliating agent) and a serum of active ingredients that maximizes the potential of the creams and the mask (ingredients: extracts of propolis, thyme, rosemary, lavender, camphor, menthol, incense, and seaweed).

• **Fair skin line**—skin with delicate blood vessels requires a particularly high level of protection against the sun and special daily nourishment. This range includes a cream (ingredients: wheat germ oil, oil of musk rose, oil of kukui, seaweed extract, allantoin, sunscreen) and a nourishing mask for weekly use.

Body and hand lotions

• **Lait Corporel Douceur (Gentle Body Milk)**—this body lotion is rich in oils and shea butter. It is enriched with extracts of propolis and *Mimosa tenuiflora* whose conditioning and protective qualities are well known (ingredients: wheat germ oil, oil of musk rose, oil of kukui, shea butter, propolis, *Mimosa tenuiflora*, seaweed extract, allantoin, fragrance).

• **Crème Raffermissante (Toning Cream)**—this cream contains extract of guaranine (a tropical creeper), rich in xanthic derivatives (caffeine and theobromine) known for their diuretic effect. It also contains a mixture of ivy, horse chestnut, and seaweed (ingredients: wheat germ oil, shea butter, guaranine, ivy, horse chestnut, seaweed).

• **Bain Moussant aux Algues (Algae Bubble Bath)**—regular use of this seaweed foam bath, rich in trace elements, gives the skin vitality and well-being (ingredients: anionic and amphoteric foaming agents of vegetable origin, seaweed extract, fragrance).

• **Bain Moussant Circulatoire (Bubble Bath for the Circulatory System)**—this foam bath contains anionic and amphoteric cleansing agents of vegetable origin. It is enriched with essential oils and plant extracts whose beneficial effects on circulation are well known (ingredients: anionic and amphoteric foaming agents of vegetable origin, extracts of seaweed, mint, cypress, lavender, red grape vine, horse chestnut).

- **Crème Mains no. 1 (Hand Cream #1)**—this oil-rich cream contains particularly effective conditioning and protective active ingredients (ingredients: plant esters, mineral oil, shea butter, oil of musk rose, oil of kukui, propolis, *Mimosa tenuiflora*, allantoin, moisturizing marine extracts).

- **Spray Fraîcheur des Jambes (Cooling Leg Spray)**—designed to refresh heavy and/or tired legs, this freshening spray consists of a very fine and penetrating emulsion that furthers the effects of the plant extracts (ingredients: apple, horse chestnut, red grape vine, camphor, menthol, eucalyptus, Melaleuca).

- **Shampooing Corps et Cheveux (Body and Hair Shampoo)**—this shampoo contains anionic and amphoteric cleansing agents of vegetable origin, a protein concentrate, and seaweed extracts.

- **Dologel**—a relaxing muscle gel that penetrates the skin easily, with a synergy of 3 percent essential oils (mint, lavender, cajeput, eucalyptus, rosemary) known for their beneficial properties for muscle relaxation.

- **Gel Harpagophytum (Harpagophytum Gel)**—*Harpagophytum procumbens* (a herbaceous plant from the deserts of Namibia) is well known for its anti-inflammatory and soothing effects on aching joints. This gel is enriched with camphor, which is also used for its decongestant effects (ingredients: camphor, Harpagophytum).

- **Huile de Massage Relaxante (Relaxing Massage Oil)**—a mixture of vegetable and mineral oils rich in esters, enriched with soothing essential oils (ingredients: wheat germ oil, mineral oil, esters of vegetable origin, essential oils).

- **Gel Chauffant (Heating Gel)**—a very fine and penetrating emulsion, this gel should be applied before intense physical activity. It stimulates the peripheral circulation, giving a feeling of warmth (ingredients: essential oils of thyme and marjoram, methyl salicylate, methyl nicotinate, extracts of seaweed and Harpagophytum).

• **Crème de Massage Camphrée (Camphore Massage Cream)**—this contains a phyto-aromatic complex with remarkably beneficial circulatory and calming properties (ingredients: water, emulsifiers, wheat germ oil, esters of vegetable extract, mineral oil, seaweed extracts, ivy, horse chestnut, red grape vine, mint, camphor).

• **Gel Douche Tonifiant aux Huiles Essentielles (Tonifying Shower Gel with Essential Oils)**—this shower gel consists of anionic and amphoteric cleansing agents of vegetable origin, a protein concentrate, and water-soluble oil. All the constituents respect the hydro-lipid balance of the epidermis. The gel is enriched with a complex of essential oils that help to tone and stimulate the muscles (ingredients: extracts of cajeput, mint, lavender, rosemary, and eucalyptus).

• **Crème de Massage aux Algues (Massage Cream with Algae)**—this cream, lightly perfumed with lemon and verbena, contains marine plant extracts rich in trace elements (ingredients: emulsifiers, wheat germ oil, esters of vegetable origin, mineral oil, fragrance).

• **Crème de Massage Minceur (Slimming Massage Cream)**—this contains vegetable extracts with the proven ability to help eliminate localized areas of excess weight (ingredients: water, emulsifiers, wheat germ oil, esters of vegetable origin, mineral oil, extracts of seaweed, ivy, and horse chestnut).

Products for dark skins
(Black is Wonderful line)

• **Ligne Eclaircissante (Lightening Line)**—this includes a serum (to be applied each morning after cleansing), a cream (to be applied each evening after removing makeup) and an exfoliating lotion (to be used three times a week).

This group is ideal for maintaining a smooth complexion or for lightening marks on the skin. It contains arbutin, a substance extracted from the leaves of the bearberry (*Arbutus uva-ursi*), a small, wild European tree. Arbutin contains natural hydroquinone, long known for its lightening effect on dark skins and age spots. While chemically produced hydroquinone has been shown to be dangerous and is now prohibited, arbutin is a natural product that does not cause irritation, since the hydroquinone it contains is of plant origin (ingredients: arbutin, symphytum, Plantago, shea butter, wheat germ, essential oils, almond oil).

• **Lait Corporel au Beurre de Karité (Body Milk with Shea Butter)**—the extraordinary traditional virtues of shea butter make this body lotion an excellent treatment for all dry skins, dark or light. It is enriched with propolis and mimosa, whose conditioning and protective properties are well known (ingredients: shea butter, mineral oil, extracts of wheat germ, propolis, mimosa, musk rose, and seaweed).

• **Gel Nettoyant Peaux Grasses (Cleansing Gel for Oily Skin)**—specially designed for dark skins, this gel is made up of plants and essential oils that exert an absorbent and anti-inflammatory action that gives the skin a clean and well-cared-for look by removing impurities (ingredients: hydroxyethyl-cellulose, propolis, ivy, watercress, arugula, rosemary, lemon, lavender).

• **Lait Démaquillant aux Germes de Blé (Wheat Germ Cleansing Lotion)**—specially designed for dark skins, this makeup remover can be used every day. It eliminates all impurities from the skin and protects the epidermis while cleansing thoroughly (ingredients: water, mineral oil, collagen, ivy, wheat germ, seaweed, fragrance).

Medical cosmetic treatments

Medical beauty treatments

I think they're just fine—for other people. I am an enthusiast of all natural and anti-aging beauty care. I am interested in everything that improves the skin; its look, its elasticity, and its tone. I am also a believer, although not a practicing one, in the virtues of antiwrinkle injections. And lastly, I have been for several years a believer in trace elements, vitamins, and food supplements.

K.L.

The aim of medical beauty treatments is to reduce the appearance of wrinkles and other facial defects (marks or scars, for example) and/or to brighten the complexion. Their advantage is that a general anesthetic is not necessary (thus avoiding possible harmful side effects) but the disadvantage is that the effects are not permanent.

Mesotherapy treatment for the face

This consists of injecting wrinkles with a nourishing and revitalizing mixture using a fine needle. Depending on the needs of the patient, the mixture may consist of vitamins, trace elements, and/or DNA extracts. Such treatments are especially suitable for fine, dry lifeless skin, or smokers' skin. The results are remarkable (healthier-looking complexion, lessening the appearance of wrinkles). However, the treatment has to be repeated at regular intervals (roughly once a month) for maximum effect.

Injections of filler

This treatment consists of injecting the product along the line of the wrinkle in order to conceal the break in the skin's surface using a very fine needle. It has been carried out for some time using collagen from cattle; this has been discontinued, however, because of the dangers linked to the appearance of mad cow disease (encephalitis, bovine spongiform). Today, it has been replaced by derivatives of hyaluronic acid, a natural polysaccharide with useful benefits for the skin, and one of the constituent elements of the subcutaneous connective tissues. The results are excellent but relatively short-lived (three to nine months depending on the dose, the site of the wrinkle, and its depth). However, the time of reabsorption varies according to the brand of the product. Numerous fillers are available worldwide. Some are completely safe; others should be avoided at all costs. It is up to the reader to carefully check the nature of the products that he or she is thinking of using.

Electrical wrinkle treatment

This consists of implanting one or several fine needles below the surface of the skin. A low-intensity electric current is then passed through the needles, encouraging the formation of collagen and filling in the wrinkle. On average, about ten treatments are required at intervals of one or two weeks, with follow-up treatments once a month to ensure lasting effects. The main benefits are in the firming of the contours of the face and improvement to fine wrinkles. This treatment is not very effective for deep wrinkles.

Botox injections

Previously there was only one method of treatment for deep horizontal wrinkles of the forehead: destruction of the muscle to prevent it from contracting. This rather drastic operation left a scar running from ear to ear, which was difficult to hide (impossible for bald people), resulting, furthermore, in a significant change in facial expression.

Today, it is possible to achieve the same effect with Botox, which "freezes" the muscle concerned; the almost painless injection goes into the muscles responsible for the formation of deep wrinkles, causing them to disappear. For a perfect result, it has to be repeated every eighteen months. The treatment must be carried out by a specially trained doctor, as the product can be dangerous in inexperienced hands. It takes only a few minutes and the patient can leave after a short rest.

Peeling

This consists of applying a chemical substance to the skin to destroy the outer layer of the skin (the epidermis) and the top layers of the dermis. This type of treatment can brighten a yellowish skin and remove age spots, small scars (such as acne scars), and wrinkles.

There are various types of "peeling" available, depending on the nature of the damage and the desired result: superficial peeling (dry ice, liquid nitrogen, fruit acids); medium peeling (trichloroacetic acid, retinoic acid, kojic acid); and deep peeling (phenol), which is reserved for very deep wrinkles accompanied by slackening of the facial tissues. Deep peeling gives the effect of a face-lift because it produces a scarring effect on the tissues.

Peeling based on fruit acids has the advantage of not being very invasive. After preparing the skin for three weeks by applying a special lotion, the doctor applies a liquid that causes a controlled desquamation (a flaking effect like sunburn). This type of peeling is an excellent method of treatment for acne scars, greasy skin, some age spots, and fine lines.

Peeling using trichloroacetic acid is slightly more invasive (the skin may itch and turn pink during the first week), but more effective. It can be used to prevent skin aging or to diminish or remove stubborn age spots, early signs of wrinkles, and skin imperfections.

The reduction of localized excess fat

Even after successful dieting, unsightly fatty deposits often remain, particularly on the stomach, arms, or legs. Cosmetic medicine has several techniques to deal with the problem.

Liposuction

This consists of sucking out the fatty tissue, usually under local anesthetic, by means of a cannula introduced into the body through a minuscule incision made in a natural groove. This method enables a precise area to be treated after weight loss (back of the knees, double chin, rounded stomach, etc.). The results are permanent.

Fat reduction by aspiration

This works on the same principle as liposuction, but is only used when very small, flattish fat deposits are removed.

Cosmetic surgery

Again, I have no problem with cosmetic surgery…for other people. Up to now I haven't needed it for myself, because I manage very well under the care of my doctor and with my own products.

What I do deplore is the way some of my acquaintances have had face-lift after face-lift and have ended up with heads that look strange and shrunken.

K.L.

We are now entering the realm of cosmetic surgery which, as we have seen with stomach operations, is never completely risk-free because of the dangers, however slight, associated with general anesthetic. That is not to say that I do not recommend it under any circumstances; merely that in certain cases it is essential to take your time during the first or the first few consultations. The patient must clearly explain what he/she wants and why, and the surgeon must explain the possible outcomes, their limitations, and the scars that will result.

That said, cosmetic surgery can perform small miracles and, even after a very localized procedure, transform someone's daily life by allowing them to come to terms with their appearance.

Facial cosmetic surgery

Face-lifts

Face-lifts (called "lifting" in French) are a surgical procedure designed to raise the facial tissues back to their original position. There are various possibilities, including the procedure that consists of repositioning skin that has moved downwards over the course of time (sagging of the facial contours, the neck, the jowls, formation of deep lines running alongside the nose); and lifting of the skin of the forehead to deal with horizontal or vertical wrinkles and crow's feet. More localized procedures are also possible (on the forehead or the neck, for example), or a complete face-lift involving the forehead, facial contours, and neck. In all cases, postoperative discomfort is inevitable (visible scars, bruising, pain), and the patient will not be "presentable" for two or three weeks. The cosmetic result is highly satisfactory in the short term and often, depending on the subject, in the medium to long term as well. Keep in mind the possibility that the procedure may need to be repeated at a later date.

Hair implants

This consists of redistributing hair from the nape of the neck (which is genetically programmed never to go bald) to bald patches. The procedure is carried out using special microsurgery instruments and requires one or more half-hour sessions depending on the degree of baldness. Today, the results of hair transplants are highly satisfactory and very natural looking, the only disadvantage being the high cost.

Cosmetic surgery of the body

It is sometimes possible to correct sagging stomachs, inner thighs, and upper arms.

There are several different techniques available to make stomachs look smoother, depending on the extent of the problem, as well as the condition of the skin, its elasticity, muscle tone, etc. Certain cases require only localized liposuction. Others (where the problem is due to loss of muscle tone) require surgery to the abdominal wall.

As for the thighs and upper arms, surgical treatment is only recommended where there is no possibility of the skin regaining its elasticity, since, when the muscle tone is very poor, there will be considerable scarring. If the sagging is not so severe, the incision can be made in the groin or armpit. Wherever possible, simple liposuction is preferable to such procedures.

Breast reduction or improvement

In certain cases, abnormally large breasts are linked to general obesity; there may be significant fatty deposits on the breasts even when the mammary gland is of normal size. Quite apart from aesthetic considerations, however, over-large breasts may cause physical problems—either back pain, neck pain, or pain between the shoulder blades (due to the breasts pulling the shoulders forward); or pain in the breasts themselves. If the breasts remain too large even after a weight loss diet, corrective surgery may be an option. There are different techniques depending on the type of incision (upside-down T-shaped, L-shaped, or I-shaped). Whatever the technique, there will be scarring and it is important to be aware of this in advance. The operation requires a short hospital stay and can transform the lives of women who have previously suffered from over-large breasts, giving them psychological benefits and a sense of well-being.

A severe weight loss diet may, in some cases, lead to a significant loss of the fatty tissue in the breasts, leading to drooping breasts ("rabbits ears"). Here also, cosmetic surgery is possible, either simply to raise the breasts or to insert implants behind the pectoral muscle in order to give the breasts a pleasing shape and size.

General medical care

There are various food supplements that can contribute to restoring general fitness. In industrialized societies it is very rare these days for lack of vitamins, mineral salts, and trace elements to lead to actual illness. Nevertheless, the systematic refinement of food (sugar, salt, flour, etc.) removes not only impurities but also a large part of the vitamins, mineral salts, and trace elements, leading to slight but chronic deficiencies. Regular use of specific food supplements (such as the Sunrex line) easily corrects such deficiencies that, although not really incapacitating, can lead to chronic fatigue.

There are also other treatments specifically for problems linked to aging; menopause for women and difficulty achieving erection for men.

Vitamins
These are essential to have in small quantities. There are two types:
- Water-soluble vitamins (all the B vitamins and vitamin C). These are found mainly in raw vegetables and fruit (the vitamins tend to be destroyed by cooking).
- Fat-soluble vitamins (A, D, E, and K). These are found in certain vegetables but mainly in fish, meat, dairy products, and their derivatives.

Mineral salts
Small quantities of sodium, potassium, calcium, phosphorus, magnesium, and chlorides are necessary for the smooth functioning of the body. A reasonably balanced diet ensures a sufficient intake of mineral salts without, as a rule, the need for supplements. Keep in mind that fish is a very good source of mineral salts.

Trace elements
Infinitesimal quantities of these substances (iron, iodine, zinc, copper, fluoride, selenium, etc.) need to be present in the body. Seafood such as fish and shellfish are an excellent source of trace elements.

Antioxidants

The phenomenon of oxido-reduction, which takes place inside the cells, is at the root of the aging process. This is particularly true for skin cells, which are the most exposed to oxidation agents. To combat this phenomenon, antioxidants are used where possible as a general treatment and also, in localized form, in "anti-aging" cosmetic products. The two principal antioxidants are vitamin C (ascorbic acid) and vitamin E.

Vitamin C protects against free radicals, which cause the skin to age by attacking the hydration of the epidermis. They multiply rapidly when the skin is damaged by such things as pollution or exposure to sun. In addition, vitamin C stimulates the production of collagen. It is present in citrus fruit, kiwifruit, and strawberries but also in pumpkin, cabbage, or fennel, preferably eaten raw, as heat destroys some of the vitamin C.

As for vitamin E, in addition to its antioxidant action, it possesses the ability to help water settle in the epidermis. Vegetable oils (sunflower, rapeseed, groundnut, and olive) all contain a certain amount, as do margarine and dried fruit.

D.H.E.A.

For some time the media has been showing great interest in a hormone that is supposedly a real fountain of youth. Numerous virtues are attributed to it, such as rejuvenation, weight loss, prevention of cancer, heart disease, Alzheimer's, etc. The hormone in question is dehydroepiandrosterone, a steroidal hormone produced in the suprarenal glands. The body begins to produce this hormone from the age of six or seven, reaching the highest level of production at about twenty-five. Thereafter, the rate of production decreases by about 2 percent per year.

At present there is fierce debate about the beneficial effects of D.H.E.A., with some scientists maintaining that insufficient trials have been carried out on humans to be certain that there are no dangers, and that there is insufficient proof of its efficacy where aging is concerned. (It owes its reputation mainly to tests carried out on rats and mice, during the course of which a reduction in the risk of cancer, obesity, and diabetes was observed.) According to different results with humans, D.H.E.A. appears to have a modest positive effect on bone density and increased libido, but mainly in women over sixty-five, who also show an improvement in skin texture (but with accompanying growth of facial hair).

If you wish to undergo D.H.E.A. treatment, medical supervision is essential. Your doctor will need to determine your existing level of D.H.E.A. to determine your needs.

Hormone replacement therapy during menopause

Although it cannot be prescribed to all women, particularly not those with a family history of breast cancer, hormone replacement therapy has revolutionized the lives of many menopausal women. Menopause refers to the period when the ovaries cease to produce hormones; the treatment consists of administering, by means of a patch, lotion, or pills, the lacking hormones.

Hormone replacement therapy has proved efficacious for all problems normally linked to menopause. It is particularly effective in preventing hot flushes and in keeping the vaginal tract lubricated, but also guards against skin aging, cardiovascular disease, and osteoporosis. Where hormone treatment is impossible or is not desired, treatment through food supplements can provide good results, using soy, yams, and sage (Menoestro, Sunrex laboratories).

The treatment of erectile disfunction

A substance that has been around for a few years, sildenafil (marketed under the name of Viagra) has made it possible to treat many problems associated with virility. It relaxes the muscles surrounding the areola of the erectile tissue of the penis and is therefore able to treat problems relating to erection in patients suffering from arterial lesions, which make erection difficult. The medication has to be taken about an hour before sexual activity. Contrary to what has been occasionally written, Viagra is not in itself dangerous, as long as it is not abused; it is recommended for use no more than once a day and the contraindications should be respected.

Another product, apomorphine chlorhydrate (marketed under the name of Uprima), works by stimulating part of the brain (the hypothalamus), which in turn stimulates the sexual organs.

For those who are wary of such products, there is an alternative therapy that can be taken in the form of a food supplement: *Tribulus terrestris*, known for its stimulant effect both generally and on the sexual function (Forman, Sunrex laboratories).

Stress management

In its general sense, stress is anything that attacks the body physically (accidents, extreme cold, extreme heat, etc.) or psychologically (bereavement, divorce, extreme fear, etc.). By extension, the unexpected shifts and changes of everyday life, such as aggressive behavior by other people, family disputes, etc. are regarded as stressful events.

Some people are more susceptible than others to stressful events and their bodies react by malfunctioning, thus bringing on various problems, more or less serious, or even psychosomatic illnesses. They are quite real and as physical as any other illness. Certain stomach ulcers, irritable bowel syndrome, or even some cancers can be brought on by the unconscious response of the sufferers to stress and conflict.

The greater a person's sensitivity, the greater the risk of stress-related illnesses. Nevertheless, in the vast majority of cases, stress does not have such serious consequences: the people concerned suffer from functional problems, meaning their bodies are not damaged but they start to malfunction. They complain of pains, spasms, a general feeling of malaise, palpitations, etc. even when the results of medical examinations are normal.

There is also such a thing as positive stress, stressful obligations that make us work harder and get on in life.

Alternative therapies

Conventional medicine has an array of tranquilizers, neuroleptics, and antidepressants to treat stress. These are effective but not without side effects and sometimes give rise to problems that lessen their effectiveness. Natural methods can also be very helpful in treating such disorders.

Some of the natural methods, which have proved to be effective in stress treatment, include acupuncture, applications of clay and mud (in thermal or thalassotherapy spas or by self-application), auriculotherapy (stimulation of pressure points in the ear), reflexology (stimulation of pressure points in the foot), homeopathy, and relaxation. But it is treatment with plants (phytotherapy), trace elements, vitamins, and mineral salts that provides the best and longest-lasting results.

Giving up smoking

Why smoke?

My father used to smoke fat cigars and my mother enjoyed American, English, or Turkish cigarettes (I forget which). I myself have never smoked—I can't see the point. I tried it, of course, but it didn't do anything for me. What's more, it seems to me that to be constantly carrying around a pack of cigarettes and a lighter, and having to find somewhere to dispose of the ash, is a completely unnecessary source of irritation. Nevertheless, I completely accept that those around me smoke, even if I don't approve of it.

K.L.

There is no point in going into what everybody already knows; let me merely repeat that tobacco is a poison and a major contributing factor to numerous serious illnesses, first and foremost cardiovascular disease and cancer (particularly of the lung and throat).

Tobacco contains several poisons, essentially tar and nicotine. The first builds up deposits inside the respiratory tract, causing irritation and congestion; this is what eventually leads to diminished lung capacity and cancer. The second causes dependency so that, when you stop smoking, the reduced levels of nicotine in the blood can cause problems such as irritability, insomnia, binge eating, etc.

Despite all these problems, it is never too late to give up smoking, even at the expense of putting on a few pounds.

There are two main ways to give up smoking: medicinal and physical. There are also psychological methods such as hypnosis, which can be used alone or in association with other techniques. Group psychotherapy is also used, in much the same way as it is for giving up alcohol.

None of these methods are infallible. Everyone has to find the one that works best for them but, in all cases, firm resolve and conviction are essential. To give yourself the best chances you must:

- Start at a time when things are relatively calm psychologically, such as during vacation time.
- Give up alcohol too, at least at the beginning.
- Avoid spicy food.
- Eat plenty of fruit rich in vitamin C (oranges, clementines, lemons, kiwis, etc.).
- Drink plenty of water.

The most essential element in the battle to quit smoking, however, is willpower.

Techniques to help quit smoking

You can try:

- Allopathy, which consists of patches or nicotine gum. The aim is to help the smoker give up by progressively lowering the amount of nicotine in the blood (the patches supply a progressively lower nicotine content), and thus minimize withdrawal symptoms, irritability in particular. In certain cases the patient may be offered a light tranquilizer or, even better, a plant remedy such as hawthorn, which has sedative properties. Furthermore, a medication hailed as a "miracle cure" was recently launched but it is too early to say how effective it will be.
- Homeopathy also has possible solutions: a homeopathic doctor can have a pharmacist make up diluted homeopathic versions of tobacco from one of your cigarettes.
- Different physical techniques can be used, either alone or in conjunction with allopathy or homeopathy. These include acupuncture and methods derived from it, such as auriculotherapy (injections or positioning of semipermanent needles at certain points on the ear or a wire stimulating the relevant points) or electric stimulation of the points with a portable device.

All these techniques give satisfactory results in the short term; the problem is the long term. The difficulty is basically to resist temptation and not backslide, seeking solace in tobacco when life gets tough. There remains the possible risk of weight gain.

Sleep—the ally of fitness

My sleep

I have always slept relatively well, especially in planes, cars, and trains. This is because I never drive. These days I sleep soundly for seven hours at a time, and I am rarely awakened by disturbances. If necessary, I am capable of fitting in five to fifteen minute naps, which are just as deep as my nighttime sleep and which leave me refreshed and full of energy.

When I was on my diet, and even now, I sometimes fall asleep dreaming of the next day's breakfast; my yogurts, my tea, and my whole wheat toast.

K.L.

Although it's difficult to explain exactly why, there is no doubt that sleep is vital. A good, tranquil sleep, in a relatively cool atmosphere, guarantees that you will wake up refreshed and is one of the main ways to feel good during the day.

Sleep allows the metabolism to slow down, giving energy to the body, while dreaming releases mental tension. On average, each individual needs eight hours of sleep for every period of twenty-four hours, with some people requiring less and some more. Interestingly, the amount of sleep needed reduces with age.

Consult your doctor!

Several million people take a sleeping pill every evening in order to go to sleep. If you are one of these people, don't go cold turkey (some remedies are addictive and must be given up gradually: sudden cessation can also cause insomnia to rebound). Start by consulting a doctor who believes in natural remedies, and who will be able to advise you on the speed with which you should replace your pills by more gentle or natural methods.

Sometimes the lack of refreshing sleep is due to problems that occur while you are asleep, particularly sleep apnea (repeated cessation of breathing). If the doctor suspects such problems he can order screening tests to determine the appropriate treatment. Another possibility is that insomnia (or conversely, excessive sleeping) can be a warning sign of depression.

Some essential rules for a good night's sleep

Learn to recognize your ideal bedtime (everyone has their own cycles, indicated by simply feeling tired, yawning fits, difficulty in keeping your eyes open, etc.). Go to bed as soon as you feel sleepy—even if it means going to bed before or after your spouse—or alternatively wait for the next cycle to begin (one and a half to two hours later) before going to bed. If sleep does not come, don't waste time worrying about it; get up and engage in some peaceful activity until you feel sleepy again. If you have trouble falling asleep, try these techniques:

- Avoid over-large meals, alcohol, and stimulants (tea or coffee) in the evening. After dinner stick to herbal teas or a cup of hot milk.
- Protect your bedroom from surrounding noise. Keep it well ventilated and not too hot, preferably not over 64°F. Choose a bed that's not too hard and not too soft, with light covers and a fairly flat pillow.
- If possible, take a little gentle exercise before going to sleep; the best preparation for sleep is a fifteen- or thirty-minute walk.
- On the other hand, it is important to avoid any strenuous exercise, either physical or mental. If you are particularly tense you can try taking a bath with scented oils every two or three days.
- For those who experience particular difficulty in getting to sleep or who suffer from chronic insomnia, various techniques have proved effective: relaxation, acupuncture, auriculotherapy, phytotherapy, or homeopathy.

Overcoming fatigue

One of the great evils of our time, fatigue is often the result of insufficient or insufficiently refreshing sleep, but it can also result from overstimulation of the senses (particularly background noise such as television, radio, traffic, public transportation, car travel) and the stress of daily life.

But fatigue may also be the result of an inappropriate diet: the excess of or lack of vitamins, minerals, metals, proteins, fats, and carbohydrates can cause hormone imbalance and digestive problems leading to a buildup of toxins and metabolic problems. This wears out the internal organs and the bone and muscle structure prematurely and causes fatigue and aging of the cells.

- Physical fatigue arises when the body fails to eliminate its waste products (lactic acids) in a satisfactory way, either because the muscles are overused or not sufficiently strong. Normally a good night's sleep deals with the problem; if tiredness persists for several days it may be necessary to reduce activity levels for a while and to turn to more drastic methods such as rest cure, massage, baths, acupuncture, etc.

- Mental fatigue (particularly problems with memory) can be linked to a phosphorus deficiency. Wheat germ, egg yolk (in moderation), mushrooms, fish and shellfish, barley, lentils: these are some of the foods that can help to make up for this deficiency. Remember also that phosphorus is assimilated more easily when taken with manganese (found in Brazil nuts, almonds, barley, whole wheat, spinach, and groundnuts).

- Psychological fatigue is the result of a prolonged period of physical and/or mental fatigue. This can lead to depression, particularly if the person concerned tries to continue as normal with the aid of stimulants instead of taking a break to let body and mind repair themselves. This gradually wears out the endocrine system and leads eventually to a state of general exhaustion. If you find yourself in this situation, consult a doctor who will, if necessary, suggest a psychological treatment (psychotherapy), medication (for a short period), or a plant-based treatment (phytotherapy). Alternatively he may suggest acupuncture or homeopathy, relaxation, or a treatment of trace elements (magnesium and selenium).

But whatever your preferred treatments may be, you should on no account allow your fatigue to become chronic. Take your life in both hands and consult your doctor!

A little exercise for total fitness

Exercise

As a child I always did a lot of exercise, especially biking, as this is the simplest way to get around in northern Germany. In addition I worked out regularly and danced a great deal. Today, I exercise every other day in my gym, starting with a few stretching exercises, then moving on to the treadmill. I do use weights but not a lot. My aim is to maintain my strength and suppleness and to feel fit. But it's important to me that my clothes hang well, so I have to be careful; you shouldn't work out too much if you want a jacket to hang perfectly.

K.L.

We are often unaware that our bodies were built for action and that it is essential for our internal organs to be massaged by movement to keep them from going slack and starting to malfunction. Even the brain and nervous system require the body to ensure a sufficient supply of oxygen for them to function effectively.

Fifteen minutes of exercise every day is enough to get fit again: if you stick to it you will be rewarded by increased calm and energy throughout the day. Join a gym, take up yoga or some other gentle type of physical activity (tai-chi for example) that focuses on breathing. Oxygen acts as the body's fuel, so exercising without getting plenty of air into your lungs means that you are forcing your engine. In other words, even if you are building up your muscles, you are wearing out your body.

Do not be impatient for results, especially if you have not exercised for some years, and allow yourself to get over the aches and pains you may experience at the beginning. You will quickly notice a real improvement to your general state of health, both physical and mental. Your blood circulation will improve and your body will become more toned. Your figure will benefit in every respect; more elegant, more supple, lighter. Fatigue will be a thing of the past, as will back pain. It's not exaggerating to state that 80 percent of back pain stems from avoidable muscle weakness. Posture also plays an important role in the incidence of this problem that affects three out of five people. Before beginning a program of gym work, consult a doctor to have your blood pressure, cardiac rhythm and respiration checked.

Although a minimum of fifteen minutes per day is necessary for the exercise to be really effective, the final result depends on keeping it up. Do not let your good resolutions slip for any reason (such as a holiday); stick to your daily routine wherever you are. If worst comes to worst, replace your daily exercises by a forty-minute walk. On the other hand, never push yourself too hard; if you experience any pain, stop and rest.

Learn to breathe

If you have not exercised for some years, you will no doubt be unaware of how to breathe to full capacity. Here are two simple ways to improve your breathing.

- Several times a day (twice in a row, morning, noon, and evening, gradually building up to more) stop, breathe in deeply, hold your breath, breathe out slowly, wait for a few minutes with your lungs empty, then take a deep, slow breath.
- With your chin lowered towards your chest and the top of your head stretched up to the sky, breathe in slowly, while forcing yourself to lower and relax your shoulders. Then breathe out slowly, letting your head fall backwards, while raising your shoulders to your ears. Do this exercise first thing in the morning and last thing at night, gradually increasing the number of breaths in and out.

Warming up

Warm-up exercises are essential before every exercise session. If you overuse your muscles when cold you risk a strained muscle.

- In a standing position with feet apart, raise your arms above your head. With palms together, straight above your head, stretch your whole body upwards from the hips. Place your arms in front of you, bending the knees, then lean forward and throw your arms out behind you. Bring your arms round in front, straighten your knees, then stand up again, throwing your arms backwards. Repeat this exercise 3 times to begin with, gradually increasing to about 10 times.

- Another warm-up exercise: in a standing position with feet apart, stretch your arms above your head in a straight line with your body and put your palms together. Stretch your whole body upwards from the hips. Keeping your arms in this position and your back and legs straight, lean forward at a right angle to your body. Hold the position. Roll your back from right to left and from left to right. Let your chest and arms fall forward loosely and stretch downwards, while keeping your legs straight. Throw your arms between your legs, stretching backwards, then stand up straight again. Do 3 sets.

Shoulder exercises

The trapezius muscles situated at the top of the shoulders tend to accumulate tension and to harden, leading to exhausting pain.

- In a standing position, with feet slightly apart and back straight, raise the shoulders towards the ears, then bring them back to their original position. (5 times)
- In the same position, move the shoulders forward (keeping the back straight) then backwards. (5 times)
- Still in the same position, make a circular movement with your shoulders from front to back, then repeat the same movement from back to front. (5 times)

Bust exercises

If you really want to change the look of your breasts, you will need cosmetic surgery. To tone them, sprinkle them with cold water every morning and perform the following exercises:

- In a standing position, with the back straight, staring at a point level with your eyes, squeeze your hands and palms tightly together on a level with your neck and mouth. Leave hands pressed together for ten seconds. Relax. (5 times)

- In a standing position, with arms crossed, grip the opposite forearm, alternately pushing and pulling. (5 times)

Exercises to make the shoulders more supple

- In a standing position, legs wide apart, feet pointing outwards, arms out to the sides, bend your wrists so that your fingers point upwards; then make circular movements with your arms, first forward then backwards. (5 times)
- In a standing position, legs wide apart, feet pointing outwards, stretch your arms out to the sides, with palms facing upwards and without bending the elbows. Push the arms upwards as if pushing the air away.
- The same exercise but with palms facing downwards and pushing downwards.
- In a standing position, feet apart, place the right hand on the right shoulder and the left hand on the left shoulder. Put your elbows together then push them forwards and upwards. Raise as high as possible. Push the elbows downwards again and finish by pulling them to each side of the body, while keeping the back straight. (5 times, then 10)
- In a standing position, with legs apart, feet apart and facing outwards, and fists clenched, cross, uncross and recross your arms in front of you like a pendulum swinging from the top of the back. (10 times)
- In a standing position, feet apart, knees slightly bent, arms hanging down straight, palms facing the floor, raise the arms backwards. (10 times)
- In a standing position, feet slightly apart, arms hanging down and bent at the elbow, fists clenched, bring fists up towards the chest. With fists still clenched, open arms out in front of you. (10 times)

Exercises for the waist and hips

- In a standing position, legs apart, back straight, stomach and buttocks tucked in, knees slightly bent and arms stretched out in front of you, move your arms one over the other in a scissor movement. (10 times)
- In a standing position, feet apart, back straight, raise your hands to touch the back of your head. Then lean from one side to the other, bending only from the waist. (10 times each direction)
- The same exercise rotating the upper body, but this time bending your arms and placing your fingertips on your shoulders. (10 times each direction)
- In a standing position, feet slightly apart, arms out to the side and bent at the elbows, touch your left knee with your right elbow, leaning forward from the waist. Repeat with your right knee and your left elbow. (10 times)
- Lie on your left side, stretching out your left arm beneath your head. Keep your feet, waist, and arm in a straight line. Raise your right leg, keeping it straight and do 10 scissor movements in an up and down direction. Repeat on the other side.

Exercises for the "stomach" and abdominal muscles

- Lie on your back on a hard surface and bend your knees as you lift them. Stretch your arms above your head and force the small of your back down onto the floor. Hold for a few seconds. (10 times)
- Lie flat on your back with your arms by your sides, palms facing downwards. Bend your knees and lift up the upper half of your body until your hands touch your ankles. (5 times)
- Same position but this time raise your knees to your chest. (5 times)
- Lie on your back, knees bent together, feet slightly apart, hands crossed behind your head. Raise the upper part of your body by lifting your shoulders and part of your back. Relax back down. (5 times)
- Same position but feet closer together. Raise your left leg, bending the foot backwards and raise the upper body towards the foot,

without letting the foot move. Repeat with the right leg. (5 times)

- Lie on your back with your knees bent and arms down by your side, palms facing downwards. With legs slightly apart, raise the whole body apart from the arms, feet, and shoulder blades. Then put your hands under your hips and gently raise yourself even further. Come back down slowly, starting from the top of your back.
- Lie on your back on a hard surface with your hands beneath your buttocks, palms downwards. Lift both legs, keeping them as straight as possible, while raising your neck and upper body. While the right leg stretches upwards, lower the left leg and vice versa, in an opening and closing scissor movement. (5 times)
- Lie on a hard surface with your hands behind your head. Raise the right elbow and left knee and bring them as close to each other as possible. Repeat with the left elbow and right knee. (5 times)

Back exercises

- Sit with your legs together and stretched out in front of you. Raise your arms straight above your head. Slowly lower the upper body until your hands touch your feet and your head rests on your knees. Do not force yourself, but hold the position as long as you can. At the beginning your knees will tend to bend. (3 times)
- Sit on a hard surface. With head and shoulders raised, bend your knees and seize hold of your feet with your hands. Holding your feet, lower your head and back forward, while pulling your feet towards your body in the direction of your shoulders, in the way that babies often do. (3 times)

A key word: balance

In order to maintain a level of fitness you need to try to organize your life and work and to maintain a balance between your family life, professional activities, leisure time, and various obligations. For many people who feel unwell, anxious, depressed, and tired, the main problem is simply their inability to organize their lives.

We often tend to take things at face value when they actually have some hidden cause. Thus some people complain of constant fatigue and look to medication for help. Others are miserable or depressed and turn to tranquilizers. Still others sleep badly, wake up during the night, and get up exhausted in the morning.

After carrying out a battery of tests, a doctor will sometimes discover the reason and be able to treat it. But in many cases it is simply a question of not being in tune with the demands of our lifestyles, something the doctor can do nothing about. He may be able to alleviate the symptoms or even get rid of them completely but, as soon as the treatment stops, the problems will return. Treatment of the symptoms can only throw a veil over the problems, not cure them.

This shows us that circumstances lead patients to adopt a lifestyle that isn't right for them, or that used to work but no longer does. The body and the mind then react in protest. For example, someone may be in an unfulfilling job, his colleagues exasperate him, he can no longer stand his spouse…but instead of acting, he takes tranquilizers and waits for things to improve…or to die of old age.

In a situation like that, you should react, open your eyes, make an effort to understand the true causes of your unhappiness. It may seem easier to ignore the problem, rather than negotiating ways of improving or eliminating it; this is a question of individual temperament and everyone must follow their own judgement. Of course, it can be difficult and painful to change jobs or separate from a spouse, but burying your head in the sand is not the answer. Everything has its price; happiness and fitness are no exception.

Positive thinking

What is the point of moaning and making yourself sick just because you are annoyed? When confronted with a difficulty, accept the situation calmly and try to deal with the problem (or the catastrophe). Once you accept that there is no point in railing against events over which you have no control, you will have taken an important step towards serenity. That doesn't mean you should become completely fatalistic, because that would lead to indifference and inactivity. On the contrary, you should react instantly, without wasting time bemoaning your fate, and find the best solutions to your problems.

Once you have surmounted the worst of your difficulties, stand back and consider whether the cause may have lain in your attitude. You may be able to learn a lesson for the future and mend your ways.

You'll find this life philosophy helpful in so many situations, from the smallest annoyances to the most serious catastrophes.

A fulfilling job

Work

People say I'm a workaholic, but for me work is not work because I do what I love. Once I begin to feel that I have had enough of one activity, I go on to another one, which refreshes me. With fashion and the things that stem from it—my photo studios, the publishers and bookstore that I run with Gerhard Steidl and various other things—I am never bored. On the contrary, I am both happy and grateful with all my activities. It goes without saying that this can only work with ruthless organization. I chose the people around me with great care and they all know what I expect of them. I would be very annoyed if time were wasted because of poor organization, for there is so much to be done, listened to, watched, read, drawn, written. There is no boredom, only boring people, who aren't interested in anything.

K.L.

To feel really fit and in shape, it's essential to have a job you enjoy and find interesting. How many people literally lose their health because of their work? In many cases, when their job doesn't interest them, they end up feeling like it's a chore, and then eventually a daily assault. Their body reacts to the assault with problems, one of which is a falling out of shape, mentally and physically.

Of course, not everyone is meant to hold important jobs, and it is possible to find satisfaction in all kinds of jobs, on the condition that you personally chose it, enjoy it, and derive personal satisfaction from it. If that is not the case, change your job if you can; the result will be worth any difficulties you may encounter. If it is not possible, compensate for your frustration by taking up outside interests. It doesn't matter what they are, as long as you enjoy them and feel fulfilled.

The virtues of organization

Staying fit requires a balanced lifestyle and balance, in turn, requires a certain regularity in life.

Don't let your free time be taken up by things you don't want to do. Simplify your life. Avoid complications unless you derive some pleasure from them. In a word, don't let yourself suffer.

At home, share the chores with your spouse.

If you work too far from home and are exhausted by the commute, change jobs—or move: if you persist, depression or a stomach ulcer lie in wait. Your body will find the situation unbearable....Don't be surprised if refusing to do anything about the situation ends up making you sick!

Find time for regular exercise. You don't have to try to be a great athlete; regular walking or swimming, jogging, aerobics, or tennis will all help to keep you in shape.

Find time to do the things you enjoy.

As for family life, finding a balance there is necessary for the good of everyone. If at all possible, reserve some time every day, even if only a few minutes, to talk to your children.

In conclusion, the key is that to be truly fit, everyone must take responsibility for themselves. They must take their lives in hand and organize themselves, so that they are a part of society without feeling crushed, while benefiting from the advantages and avoiding, as much as possible, the disadvantages. This is the only way to achieve true fitness, for mental equilibrium is essential to that of the body.

Conclusion

Sometimes his shrewd eyes seemed to glaze over with unconcerned indifference, as befits a consummate dandy and a man who carries within himself something superior to the visible world.

Jules Barbey d'Aurevilly,
Du dandysme et de George Brummell

Tao that is named is not Tao. Tao that is written down is not Tao. Better to block your ears than to hear the name Tao spoken.

He who intuitively understands Taoism cannot resist substituting it with the word "dandyism." To paraphrase Cioran's aphorism: He who lives in the knowledge that he is a great saint is not a great saint.

The same goes for the concept of dandyism, which is definitely not as simple as the Larousse dictionary definition: "Style of dress and of physical attractiveness, based on refined elegance, perpetually renewed and associated with an affectation of wit and impertinence."

Dandyism is an indefinable state of mind, characterized by a determined striving for absolute harmony between the individual and his surroundings and, in one's appearance, by the external signs of this quest.

As is often the case, the world has misunderstood dandyism and, mistaking the effects for the causes, tends to regard dandies as hopeless eccentrics, light and frivolous creatures, superficial and smug individuals, high on themselves, and completely uninterested in the rest of humanity.

By making such assumptions, society deprives dandyism of its spiritual element and reduces the dandy to a ridiculous puppet. Take the swooning and conceited serving stretched out over seven chairs, overturned like a jumble of bowling pins in the gardens of the Palais-Royal, as illustrated by Paul Gavarni; this is not a dandy but rather his "likeness," lacking the gravity that distinguishes alpha from omega. If, in the first instance, dandyism is all about concern for appearance, in the final analysis it is an act of rejection of the world and of oneself in the most penitent of garb: that of elegance. He becomes fainter and fainter, a silhouette marching in the opposite direction from the emerging world, with his walking stick, like a periscope, pointing towards the oblivion of the continent that Apollinaire, the Omega dandy, implored.

This is the way the world is going and it is not easy for those who still practice dandyism to continue to stand firm and maintain a climate in which they can survive. It is only by making countless concessions to the world that the ultimate dandies have succeeded in maintaining the basic essentials of their raison d'être: a great liberty and originality of thought. These two characteristics of the spirit of dandyism obviously influence their behavior, and their lifestyle is characterized by originality. Eccentric dress is strictly optional, so it could be said that some are only dandies in principle whereas others, who dress more showily, are "complete" dandies. The pursuit of this philosophy is not without problems and is often greeted by antipathy, arrogance, or provocation, or is even regarded as antisocial. Dandies have to put up with all sorts of irritations and insults. Often criticized and sometimes jeered at, they are in a perpetual state of conflict with themselves—torn between what they are and what they would like to be—trying to achieve harmony with their ideal.

The torment that governs the life of a dandy, can only find expression in comedic drama.

No tears on the surface!
Play the mysterious martyr
Hide your curious soul
Each time you brush past them

At the sound of sorrowful music
Pour forth your anxious dream
No tears on the surface!
Play the mysterious martyr

Be silent until death!
The true melancholic is silent
And conscience has eyes
To cry at every moment
No tears on the surface!

This injunction from Maurice Rollinat, dandy and tragic author of *The Neuroses*, follows the rule of asceticism as laid down by Oscar Wilde: "Like the good Francis of Assisi, I am married to poverty; but in my case it is an unsuccessful union." "The Ballad of Reading Gaol," a true work of black humor, carries at its heart the seeds of apparent frivolity, such as the lily the protagonist carries down Piccadilly, and the insults hurled at the decor of his hotel bedroom in Alsace: "I fought a duel to the death with the wallpaper."

The spirit of dandyism swings between the two extremes of gravity and futility. Thus Brummell, "king of fashion," broke and sick, near to death, begged the nuns in the hospice at Caen to give him a mirror, as nothing seemed more important than to check his appearance.

The frivolity of the dandy, as exemplified by Karl Lagerfeld when he says, "I want to be an elegant clotheshorse," hides, in reality, an inflexible determination to subjugate his body and to mold it into what his spirit wants.

For the dandy, real elegance is the fruit of a mystical battle against the material world, the run of the mill, and the conventional: "In literary cafés and in my most affected bearing, I maintain that I am a sorrowful man. Are people surprised by my confidence? My elegance is my leprosy; this walking stick is my discipline. This hand which you say is beautiful has never been touched by another. It has only received peremptory waves." (Jean Paral, *Entretiens du Café de Flore—lettres Alchimiques*)

My friend Karl Lagerfeld undertook his metamorphosis as one undertakes religion, after meditating long and hard on his decision. He stuck firmly to his self-imposed discipline and I think that today he is happy to have reached his goal. I think that now he is able to relax the way you would after returning home from a long and difficult journey, something that is poetically expressed in the following sentences: "Our silhouettes superimposed themselves exactly on top of one another until they achieved metaphysical unity and we were silent…for a long time and spiritedly. Since that day we have never been apart and have had one and the same face: the discreet and pale one of walk-on actors, masked by the artifice of tender and brutal colors." (Jean Paral, *Monographie d'un petit elephant mauve ou trente-six instantanés*)

In conclusion, the dandy is like the mystic in the most painful sense, because he is so unconventional. A timeless vagabond, he moves through crowds, sometimes fêted, sometimes abused, but always raising awareness and provoking the question, "What is that?"—a precursor to the philosophical "Who are we?"; the beginning of reflection on the meaning of life.

For those who think that all you need to become slim and elegant is to go on a diet and exercise, here is a final warning: *The only true elegance is that of the soul.*

Jean-Claude Houdret

Tables

Ideal weights for women according to height

Height	small Frame	medium Frame	large Frame
4'10"	92.4 – 98.6	96.4 – 107.6	104.3 – 119.5
4'11"	93.1 – 102.1	97.0 – 111.1	105.2 – 123.0
5'	95.5 – 104.5	100.3 – 113.5	108.2 – 125.4
5' 1"	97.7 – 108.0	102.7 – 117.0	110.7 – 128.9
5' 2"	101.2 – 110.4	106.0 – 19.5	114.2 – 131.3
5' 3"	103.6 – 114.0	108.5 – 123.2	116.6 – 135.3
5' 4"	107.1 – 116.4	112.2 – 126.5	120.1 – 138.4
5' 5"	110.0 – 120.1	114.4 – 131.6	123.0 – 143.2
5' 6"	113.1 – 123.2	118.8 – 135.3	127.8 – 146.3
5' 7"	115.9 – 128.0	121.9 – 139.9	130.9 – 150.9
5' 8"	120.6 – 131.1	126.5 – 143.2	135.5 – 154.2
5' 9"	123.9 – 136.2	129.8 – 147.8	138.8 – 159.1
5' 10"	128.5 – 141.7	134.4 – 52.5	143.4 – 165.0
5' 11"	133.1 – 144.8	139.3 – 155.8	148.1 – 169.0
6'	136.4 – 149.4	142.3 – 160.4	151.4 – 174.9
6' 1"	141.0 – 150.9	147.0 – 161.9	156.0 – 176.9

Ideal weights for men according to height

Height	small Frame	medium Frame	large Frame
5' 2"	111.1 – 120.3	117.3 – 131.8	131.8 – 141.2
5' 3"	113.5 – 123.9	119.5 – 134.0	127.6 – 145.2
5' 4"	117.0 – 126.3	123.0 – 136.2	131.1 – 148.5
5' 5"	119.5 – 130.2	125.4 – 140.1	133.5 – 153.1
5' 6"	123.0 – 133.3	128.9 – 143.2	137.1 – 156.4
5' 7"	125.8 – 137.9	131.8 – 48.3	139.9 – 162.4
5' 8"	130.7 – 141.2	136.6 – 152.0	145.2 – 166.1
5' 9"	133.8 – 146.1	139.7 – 156.9	148.7 – 170.7
5' 10"	138.4 – 151.6	144.6 – 161.9	153.3 – 176.0
5' 11"	143.2 – 154.7	149.2 – 165.9	158.2 – 180.0
6'	146.3 – 159.5	152.2 – 171.8	161.9 – 185.9
6' 1"	150.9 – 162.8	157.1 – 175.8	167.0 – 191.6
6' 2"	154.2 – 168.3	160.2 – 181.7	170.7 – 195.6
6' 3"	158.8 – 171.4	165.7 – 185.7	176.7 – 199.5
6' 4"	161.9 – 176.2	169.6 – 191.4	180.0 – 205.5
6' 5"	166.8 – 177.8	175.6 – 193.4	184.8 – 207.5

Postscript

Karl Lagerfeld came to dinner with me last week and during the course of the low-calorie meal (jellied gazpacho with avocado cream and crayfish tails, fillets of threadfin, boiled potatoes, mixed salad, tropical fruit salad), washed down with Diet Pepsi, he remarked to me, "I like your conclusion very much but you only talk about dandies. What about women?"

Indeed, I was so wrapped up in my subject, "How I helped Karl Lagerfeld lose weight," that I forgot about women, who are actually ever-present in my mind. Throughout the book I have been thinking of them, and my recipes, advice on cosmetics, and general advice are dedicated largely to them.

In my view, everything that applies to men also applies to women with, of course, variations according to the female physiology. Like it or not, women's lives are affected by their hormones, which are constantly changing as life passes from puberty to post-menopause via pregnancy. At each of these stages there can be specific problems, but my dietary suggestions remain valid in all periods except pregnancy (when they should be adapted).

It is fashionable in the modern world for women to be relatively slim (though not too thin), but it has not always been like that. Even today standards of beauty vary from culture to culture: African women are expected to be more rounded, Asiatic women more slender, Nordic women more well built, etc.

It is important therefore, ladies, that you should make the most of your personality, bearing in mind who you are and not forgetting that you are all different and there is no obligation to give in to pressure from the media, where singers and movie stars are shown off as "ideal women." Each one of you has the right to expect the best from yourself psychologically as well as physically. Keep my last piece of advice at the back of your mind: *Your ideal weight, ladies, is the weight at which you feel good.*

Jean-Claude Houdret

Index

The Karl Lagerfeld Diet

First published in Germany in 2002 by Steidl Verlag, Göttingen

Published in the United States in 2005 by powerHouse Books,
a division of powerHouse Cultural Entertainment, Inc.
68 Charlton Street, New York, NY 10014-4601
telephone 212 604 9074, fax 212 366 5247
e-mail: lagerfeld@powerHouseBooks.com
website: www.powerHouseBooks.com

Library of Congress Cataloguing-in-Publication Data:

Lagerfeld, Karl.
 [3-D-Diät. English]
 The Karl Lagerfeld diet / by Karl Lagerfeld and Jean-Claude Houdret ;
 interview by Ingrid Sischy.
     p. cm.
 Includes index.
 ISBN 1-57687-251-3 (pbk.)
 1. Weight loss. I. Houdret, Jean-Claude. II. Sischy, Ingrid. III. Title.
 RM222.2.L2713 2005
 613.2'5--dc22
                          2004028073

Paperback ISBN 1-57687-251-3

Separations by Steidl, Göttingen
Printing and binding by Lotus Printing, Inc.

A complete catalog of powerHouse Books and Limited Editions is available upon request; please call, write, or get slim on our website

10 9 8 7 6 5 4 3 2 1

Printed in Hong Kong